Conte

Disclaimer

This book does not provide medical advice; it is intended for informational purposes only and is based upon my opinion, experiences and research. It is not a substitute for professional medical advice, diagnosis or treatment. Never ignore professional medical advice in seeking treatment because of something you have read in this book. Always seek professional medical advice.

Dedication

This book is totally dedicated to the two most important people in my life... My 23-year-old identical twin daughters Abby and Beth! Without them this book would never have even been thought of, let alone out there now helping thousands of women go through the Menopause, with hopefully a more informed and better understanding of what will happen to their bodies and even more importantly, knowing there is hope and help out there!

With them both having pressurised full-time jobs (Abby is a Biochemist and Beth is a London Paramedic) they work tirelessly day and night, sometimes around the clock to support me. With my total lack of tech skills, from showing me how to do my first post on Instagram, to spending hours of their time uploading blogs, applying for affiliate programmes, taking flat lay photos and improving the Search Engine Optimisation of clipboardclaire.com the list is just endless! They constantly encouraged me to go with my heart and do what I always wanted to do...Help others! Even with no budget whatsoever, the girls paid for all we needed to get started, knowing that as an out of work Beauty Therapist (due to Covid-19) and being in lockdown, I had no money coming in from work at all. There were things that had to be paid for, and they did not hesitate to order them, and half the time did not tell me!

Well, we have done it girls, and I am so super proud to be your mum, a single mum yes, but an immensely proud one who knows the values I taught you shine through! You are both beautiful, lovely, kind, caring and selfless young ladies both inside and out. I truly hope that when it comes to you girls going through this menopause malarkey, you will be better informed, and it will be taught in schools as standard and not the taboo subject it has been for too many years. I am sure you cannot possibly learn anymore about it than you already have in the last year, but hey, you know my motto 'forewarned is forearmed'!

Thank you both, for all your love, hard work and total dedication with clipboardclaire.com.

Love you both more than you will ever know...

Mumma Bear XX

(aka Clipboardclaire)

Foreword

So, why did I write this help and information book? Simply, to make sure another woman does not go through the years of suffering like I did, with endless GP and Consultant appointments, barely existing and having virtually no life. I want women to be better informed and of course my favourite saying of all, that I say out loud, and far too often for my liking, with such conviction "being forewarned is forearmed" and that is so important! If only I knew then what I know now! For so many of us, years have been wasted when they should not have been, purely down to a lack of information, the menopause not being talked about, and women left suffering in silence thinking they were going mad or worst still... suicidal. In this day and age, it should not be this way and for me personally, sharing my story, makes me feel I am doing something. I have a large Menopause Help group and I listen and read hundreds of messages from women every day, asking the same questions I was asking years ago. Something has got to change! So here I am making that change, getting this book out there and getting women better informed!

My Personal Menopause Journey.

For me it was nearly 9 years ago now, that life changed, and my Menopause Journey began...

Just when you think life is becoming easier, your children are growing up, work-life is consistent and the general pressures of life have mellowed, the menopause arrives.

As much as we females know it is going to happen to us one day, nobody tells us just how hellish it can be. My personal experience did not include the usual symptoms, so I felt quite alone from the word go - I did not have any hot flushes or night sweats and hadn't previously suffered at the usual time of the month, so didn't think too much about the menopause until my GP mentioned that a blood test had come back indicating I had low oestrogen levels, which is a sign of being perimenopausal.

One night I woke up in the early hours of the morning thinking that I had rolled onto my hand in my sleep. My two fingers were so painful that I was convinced I had dislocated them. I stumbled to the bathroom half asleep and ran them under a warm tap, rubbing them gently to make the pain go away. I did not know at the time, but this was the start of my journey through the menopause and if I thought this was bad, I had a lot more coming my way over the next few years. I started to get pains in my elbows next and at times struggled to carry a handbag or carry a cup of tea. This pain gradually moved to both sides of my body, to my knees and my hips. I would have considered myself to be quite fit at 45, going to the gym 4 or 5 times a week and being able to eat what I wanted to most of the time, but during this period I struggled to walk, stand, and sit for long periods and it made my work as a Beauty Therapist almost impossible.

I was sent for countless blood tests, X-rays, and MRI scans to try and discover what it was causing my joints so much pain. I was sent to multiple Physios, GPs and Consultants and the idea of Arthritis, Fibromyalgia and Lymes Disease were thrown around quite often, but my test results always came back clear. After years of pain, I was eventually told that this joint pain was down to the menopause and the only way to get through it was by pain relief. This had not crossed my mind as I did not have the common symptoms, but the idea began to make more sense over the years whilst I developed a low mood, survived on a few hours of sleep a night, and could not remember the word I needed to finish my sentence, let alone why I'd walked downstairs and gone into the kitchen.

Nobody prepares you enough for the menopause and if someone had mentioned to me that my joint problems were linked to it, it would have saved years of investigation, wasted NHS money and sleepless nights worrying what was wrong with me. I am writing this book at the age of 53 now and although I still struggle with a bad neck, my joint problems are ok and better than they were. I have tried most medications, herbal remedies, and every support I could find on the internet. My website blog clipboardclaire.com that I launched July 2020, has helped me learn so much about the menopause with the endless research that I do for my blogs, and what I can do to improve my joint problems.

I want to tell my readers about what I was never prepared for, what I found helped me and how to get through this time in your life as a female. I know everyone suffers from different symptoms of the menopause and some are lucky enough to have very few symptoms, if any at all. Every woman's journey and experience through the menopause is different of course, and no one solution or remedy fits all. But, as a post-menopausal woman I promise you, you will get through it and I hope that with the help of this book, you will have the preparation and knowledge that lots of us ladies never had and your transition through it will be an easier, smoother and happier one.

Introduction

Originally born and bred in Berkshire, my dream as a child was always to be a Beauty Therapist, I was always looking after everyone and bossing them around as a child and often found scraping hard skin off people's feet! That was not the way my career path went for many years, as you will find out. I left school in 1994 at the age of 16, I had been offered my dream job as a Beauty Therapist, but it fell through at the last minute, leaving me pretty heartbroken. I ended up working for my friend's dad who owned a Car Repair Centre, not my plan at all, but little did I know that was where my motor trade career would begin, and one I am quite proud of today. I always had a passion for cars and over the next two decades I worked for lots of car dealerships, and then ended up in a sales job, selling advertising space to the motor trade for a local newspaper. Within a few years I landed a job at the Thames Valley Auto Trader and had a successful career being one of the 13 Field Sales Executives. I met some amazing people during my career and my knowledge of cars was huge for a female, but there was always something about being a successful female in a predominantly man's world that drove me on! I loved being part of a hugely successful team, I worked hard and partied harder, smoked when I drank and lived life to the full.

At the age of 30, I found out I was pregnant, gave up my fabulous career and moved down to Hampshire to be with my babies (yes, I was expecting twins!) dad and started a new life with him when the twins were born. Sadly, when they were 2 years old, he left, and we have never seen him since. Thrown into being a single mum, I dedicated myself to bringing the girls up single handedly. It was when they were at school that I decided to go back to college and train to be a Teaching Assistant (I helped at their village school and one of the teachers said I should go and train and get a qualification). I often saw the Beauty Therapists training and started to think about my old passion and childhood dream of being a Beauty Therapist. I could then work around the girl's school hours and term time, when it would suit me better.

Fast forward 15 years, and after struggling with debilitating menopausal joint problems, and this affecting me with my beauty work, my daughters came back home in lockdown July 2020, Abby from university (to finish her Biochemistry dissertation) and Beth for a few days off work from London Ambulance Service. They sat me down and told me that they could not bare to see me struggling anymore with my job/ work and that I should go with my heart and dream of helping others and launch a website blog! That was it, CLIPBOARDCLAIRE.COM was born during lockdown from my lounge!

I have always been hugely organized and tidy and often called Clipboard Claire because of it. This time it was no joke, we ate, slept, breathed, and worked 7 days a week for nearly a year, creating blogs, taking photos, promoting it all on social media, posting on other groups, the workload was huge. The girls worked in between their full-time jobs and every bit of time they had off.

My absolute passion, drive, and determination was to not see anyone else suffer alone with these menopause symptoms and stop wasting NHS money on endless GP and Consultant appointments, that are very often menopause related. If women only knew the signs and symptoms it would save a lot of heartache, stress and worry.

I personally hit the gym 4 or 5 times a week to keep my joints going, I drink occasionally, gave up smoking many years ago and try and eat healthily. I go to bed at a reasonable time and "try" to have me time and not work ridiculous hours, but in all honesty that is not easy when you are a woman on a Menopause Mission! I find it is the drive and determination that makes me feel that I have purpose and being single during the lockdown, means this hard work has kept me sane.

All is not lost ladies, and I hate hearing daily, that women are suffering in silence, there IS light at the end of this tunnel! It IS NOT all doom and gloom and the end of your life. It is learning to adapt and deal with the menopause the way that is best for YOU! The Menopause in general, is portrayed to be such a rubbish time. It is not, I know lots of women who have new relationships, new jobs and started to learn something new. This new chapter in our lives needs to be celebrated and embraced we need to not be so hard on ourselves. Acceptance is another big one, it is just another phase of your life and being armed with as much knowledge as possible can only ever be a good thing. Use menopause trackers (on our website) and take them to your GP who then has all the information in front of them and they can take a copy. This will get you a diagnosis quicker, and not waste as much of your time with back-and-forth appointments.

The thing that spurs me on daily, hourly even, and makes me get up in the middle of the night and write down another idea I have (and I will not remember in the morning if I do not!) is to help spread this menopause topic around the world and get it out there and talked about! There are millions of women going through this journey right now, it should be taught in schools, covered in TV programmes and talked about in

Parliament! Businesses should be helping their female workforce stay in work and support them at this time.

I also feel that if, as women we do not understand what is going on with our bodies, there is not much hope for our male population, who will certainly have no idea. We cannot expect them to be empathetic, or even interested with such a lack of information for us let alone them.

So, this is my reason and drive for writing my blogs and getting this book out there, not many people have time to read a long lengthy book, or can take it all in at once, especially men with a short attention span. All 35 symptoms of the menopause are covered in short, but informative, quick, reads, that your significant other half can read too.

I hope you find it helpful and informative and learn something from it, remember, you have got this ladies! Be strong and positive and remember, this is just a new chapter of your life, and life is for living after all!

To visit our website clipboardclaire.com

What is Menopause?

Menopause is when your periods have stopped for 12 consecutive months, but the term is often referred to and includes the years leading up to this time, and for a number of years afterwards.

Perimenopause:

The lead up to menopause is known as Perimenopause, during this stage periods become irregular and menopausal symptoms can start to appear, this stage can last for many years, but each woman is different. This stage is usually experienced between the ages of 40 – 50, but again can start much younger or older. The Oestrogen production decreases substantially and can take its toll mentally, as well as physically and emotionally. Some women do not know they are in perimenopause and experience very few, if not any symptoms, but for others it is a roller coaster of debilitating symptoms, including:

- Hot Flushes
- Weight Gain
- Sleep Issues
- Depression
- Anxiety
- Heavy Bleeding
- Vaginal Dryness
- Painful Sex
- Dry Skin
- Brain Fog
- Memory Issues

- Mood Swings

Keeping a log of your symptoms is a good way of tracking your transition through this time, using a Menopause Symptom tracker is great for your GP to recognise and diagnose menopause quickly with all the information to hand.

It is possible to have fewer symptoms if you keep to a healthy lifestyle and make any changes whilst you go through this transition period. Giving up smoking, drinking minimal alcohol, eating a healthy, well balanced diet, and taking regular exercise is key going through the menopause.

Menopause:

After 12 consecutive months of no periods, you have gone through menopause. Your ovaries have stopped working, and do not produce Oestrogen anymore. The menopause often begins between the ages of 44 – 55 years old, but the average age for this time is 51 years old, the symptoms are still similar to perimenopause, but are often not as frequent or as intense and some go altogether. Every woman's menopause experience is unique to them, and some symptoms can happen suddenly or happen over a shorter period than others. Some factors can affect the severity and duration of symptoms include, having a hysterectomy, cancer, or unhealthy lifestyle choices like smoking. Other common symptoms of menopause include:

- Urinary Tract Infections
- Difficulty Concentrating
- Sore Breasts

- Headaches
- Racing Heart
- Hair Loss
- Brittle Nails
- Dry Mouth
- Facial Hair Growth
- Reduced Libido
- Painful Joints

Post menopause:

You are classified as post menopause one year after your periods have completely stopped. Once you have gone through this transition you can be more vulnerable to heart disease and osteoporosis (bone disease). Eating a healthy diet is so important at this time, and calcium is important for your bones, to keep them healthy and strong.

The more we understand and are educated about the menopause, the easier the transition through it. Knowing what to expect and dealing with the symptoms from the start, is absolutely paramount. No one should be struggling with day-to-day life, and left feeling isolated and alone, having no where to turn. The way through this should be learning what works for you and what you can do to lessen your symptoms and still have a good quality of life. Nutrition, Exercise, and knowledge will get you through this time and there IS help out there! Whether you are lucky enough to do it all naturally with very few symptoms or you take HRT (Hormone Replacement Therapy) or change your lifestyle, there is life after menopause! It is never too late to try something different, as long as you keep self-care at the top of your list, you can live a happy and fulfilling life again.

So, do not sit and suffer, make that appointment to see your GP and discuss your options and change any bad habits to healthy ones! Be positive and remember you are stronger than you think and can achieve more than you know!

Hot Flushes

Now, I must be honest, I have never suffered with these! But if anybody has asked me about anything to do with the Menopause it has been Hot Flushes! So, I have been talking to lots of friends, carried out some research and here is what I found...

I never realised up to 80% of women get hot flushes, yes, I am in the 20% that don't! I have lots of friends that get them so severely, it makes their life a living hell. Apparently, the good news is that you do not look as hot as you feel and apparently others around you do not really notice.

It seems that nobody really knows what causes these flushes, but it seems to be down to a few factors.

When your Oestrogen levels drop or decrease your body's thermostat (called the Hypothalamus) becomes overly sensitive to even the slightest of changes and thinks your body is too warm and starts to cool you down quickly by having a Hot Flush. Stress is another big factor and low levels of Serotonin could also play a part. Lots of ladies turn to Herbal Remedies and there seem to be lots of conflicting reports as to what works and what doesn't, I think it is down to the individual and it's always worth trying to find what works for you, because everyone is different.

There are also some foods that can fight these flushes, apparently Flaxseed can dampen down the effects of falling Oestrogen levels and reduce the amount of Hot Flushes. Some say its great sprinkled over some cereal. A Mediterranean Diet can also be of massive benefit and lots of vegetables and whole grain noodles have been shown to help too.

- Coffee has been known to trigger Hot Flushes due to the caffeine elevating your heart rate and causing dehydration, which in turn intensifies those feelings. Maybe try decaf Coffee and Green Tea to help with those caffeine cravings.
- Sage... lots of research has suggested that Sage can reduce the frequency and severity of night sweats and Hot Flushes, I have some friends that takes Sage tablets but I'm told you can also drink Sage Tea or use Fresh Sage in cooking.

Keeping cool, seems to be an absolute must for lots of my friends that suffer, and they often use a fan or spray some cold water from an atomiser on their face. I have even got one friend that uses a cold gel pack on the back of her neck and swears by it. Obviously not wearing tight fitting clothes, having light cotton sheets on your bed and not having a heavy duvet, all help I am told. I also have friends that say some food such as, alcohol, coffee, spicy foods, and chocolate wreak havoc with the Hot Flushes and night sweats.

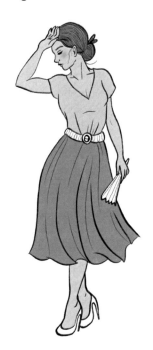

Pilates and Yoga... are another good idea and I have friends that swear by these classes. Slowing down your breathing using their techniques helps to relax the muscles, slowing the heart rate down and lowering blood pressure too.

A few other ideas tried and tested by friends are...

A fresh cup of herbal tea with 2 teaspoons of Sage can calm your flushes. Cool Max bedsheets and a very cold bedroom before you get into bed can keep night sweats away. Pillows that contain cooling gel help you to relax and sleep better.

Friends have said the following also help with Hot Flushes...

- Black Cohosh
- Ginseng
- Red Clover
- Evening Primrose Oil

No two women are alike and neither are the ways their bodies react to hot flushes. Keep trying different methods and remedies until you find one that works for you! Just remember, this time will pass!

> This is a brilliant book which highlights for women of all ages about the transition in life she will face. Knowing about the perimenopause/menopause and being prepared is really important for everyone, especially empowering women with the knowledge that they can then discuss with the GP early on if they are not coping with their symptoms.
>
> -Dr Nighat Arif
> (NHS GP,
> Resident Doctor on BBC breakfast and ITV
> this morning)

Night Sweats and Cold Flushes

Night Sweats

Night sweats are very common during the Menopause (over 75% of women say they have suffered with them) they can frequently disturb your sleep and are a related symptom to Hot Flushes during the daytime. These symptoms are the most common ones experienced by women going through the Menopause and can be very debilitating if they cause you a total lack of sleep. They become more noticeable at night because you are in bed and sleeping (or trying to get sleep) and you are not able to take any action if you feel one coming on. Lots of women wake up drenched in sweat, whilst others do not seem to be affected by the sweating at all. Like Hot Flushes, night sweats are extremely unpredictable, there is no particular time of the night they can happen, and the number of night sweats suffered can vary from one night to the next.

What causes Night Sweats?

Due to the Oestrogen levels falling during Menopause, the body's thermostat (Hypothalamus) is thrown into confusion, no-one is entirely sure why, but it is thought the hypothalamus gets confused into thinking that the body is over-heating. It starts to make the body sweat to cool down, hence the usual body response with heat, the skin reddens, the sweat glands start working and excessive sweating begins.

What can we do to help with Night Sweats?

- Have a cool bedroom, night sweats are made worse if the bedroom is warm, do not have the heating on either.
- Avoid stressful situations if possible, any upset can add to adrenaline, this makes the sweat glands work harder.
- Smoking can make night sweats worse.
- Avoid hot drinks before bedtime.
- Avoid hot and spicy food.
- Drink plenty of fluid during the day, keeping hydrated.
- Have a lower tog duvet.
- Wear light, cool clothing.
- Have a cool shower before bedtime.
- Have a fan on all night.

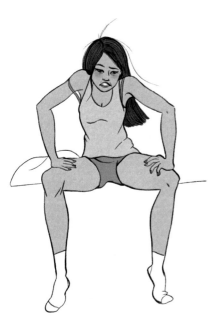

- Lose weight and exercise regularly.
- Cooling Sprays- or cooling Gels can help.
- Cool Bedding and Pillows – Can keep the body cooler and temperature down. My friends absolutely rave about this bedding from Marks and Spencer for keeping them cool at night!

What can I take to help with Night Sweats?

- HRT - Your GP may suggest taking this to see if it helps, with the drop in Oestrogen levels, HRT can help with hot flushes and night sweats. Some GPs' may recommend other medication such as a mild antidepressant.

- Yoga or Tai Chi – may help, with their relaxing techniques. Taking any regular exercise can help too especially with stress.
- CBT – Cognitive Behaviour Therapy, can improve low mood and anxiety, it is a talking therapy that works for lots of women.

Supplements that can help with Night Sweats

- Valerian – For relief of sleep disturbance and anxiety.
- Flaxseed – can reduce night sweats.
- Vitamin B – Aids sleep.
- Vitamin E – Good for Insomnia.
- Magnesium – Great for a good night sleep.

What works for one does not always work for another, we are all unique, but using a sleep tracker can determine the best remedies that help you. If you are suffering too much with sleep deprivation these will help your GP work out what medication might work for you.

Cold Flushes

Most people have heard of Hot Flushes but lots of women suffer with Cold Flushes too. It is a cold, shivery and tingling feeling, that can leave you pale and feeling shaky. Often, they do not last long and are only momentary, but effect 100's of women every day. Cold Flushes work the same as Hot Flushes, the fluctuating hormones during the menopause cause the hypothalamus (the body's thermostat) to be all over the place. Sometimes hot and sometimes cold, it is the lack of Oestrogen that plays havoc with our body temperature, either over heating us or making us freezing cold.

Other reasons for having Cold Flushes during Perimenopause and Menopause

- Changes to your Period cycle.
- Fatigue and feeling tired.
- Weight gain.
- Thinning hair
- Vaginal dryness.
- Mood swings.

Other Mood Disorders that cause Cold Flushes

Anxiety attacks are another symptom of the menopause, and lots of mood disorders can contribute to Cold Flushes too. Panic attacks are another major symptom going through the Menopause, the body releases adrenaline and other chemicals that trigger the body's 'fight or flight' reaction. This can affect your ability to control your body temperature.

What to do if you are having a Cold flush

There is very little you can do initially but wait for it to pass, once it has and your temperate re-regulates itself you should warm up. A few things you can do to lower the likelihood of having Cold Flushes are;

- Move around during the episode, do not stand still.
- Add a few layers whilst you are having a cold flush.
- Try yoga or deep breathing techniques to try and find ways to relax.

If you are concerned about cold flushes always go and speak to your GP, especially if they are affecting your daily life or you are sleeping badly. Again, tracking as much information about them as possible will help your GP to recommend any treatment.

" By the time I was 14, I was post menopausal.

Being told you are too young to be going through the menopause is not an acceptable answer! It will and does happen earlier as it did with me.

Your book is marvellous. It's great that every symptom has its own chapter so if you are feeling a certain way you can look a symptom up quickly. It's definitely a great book for partners to read as it is so simply but effectively put. I feel this book would be massively suitable to be in workplaces!

- Hayley Cockman
(Diagnosed as post-menopausal at 14). "

Joint Pain

For anyone that knows me, they know THIS is my thing! If there is one symptom of the Menopause that has been debilitating and crippled me, its joint pain! If you have read 'My Menopuase Journey' blog, you too will know how much of an effect this has had on my life. So, looking into it has been one of my easier blogs to write.

I never realised just how many women suffer with painful joints, stiffness when moving and generally 'hurt' all over. I know from all the information I have read and endless searching for a solution for myself, I have found that it's just another Menopause issue down to the diminishing Oestrogen levels and not just an age related issue. Oestrogen plays an important role in maintaining joints and keeping our bones healthy, but it is uncertain how it does this, but is thought to minimise the swelling around the joint.

Some key points to remember to aid joint pain are;

- Keep hydrated - dehydration contributes to joint pain.
- Most common joints effected by Menopause are – fingers, wrists, neck, shoulders, knees, and hips.
- Maintain a healthy weight – less pressure on the joints.
- Exercise – low impact exercises such as yoga, swimming, and biking.
- Eat a balanced diet – including lots of nutrients, including vitamin D and Calcium.
- Take anti-inflammatory Medication – Ibuprofen can help.

- See your GP if it becomes unbearable – My GP prescribed Naproxen and it helped me.
- Physiotherapy – This can be a great help in keeping you mobile.
- Alcohol and smoking – Alcohol depletes the body of water which increases inflammation causing joint pain and smoking has been found to increase sensitivity making pain worse too.
- Avoiding stress – this can have a negative effect on your joints as high quantities of the hormone cortisol are released.
- Poor posture – this puts extra pressure on your joints and limits your range of motion and makes it harder for the muscles to take the load off your joints.

Foods that can ease joint pain;

- Omega-3-rich-foods - contain lots of oils and have a positive effect on inflammation. (Salmon, Sardines, Tuna, Almonds, Chia seeds, Soybeans)
- Antioxidant-rich-foods – these foods have powerful antioxidants that reduce inflammation. (Raspberries, Broccoli, Peppers, Blueberries, Cherries)

Lots of fruit and vegetables reduce inflammation, so keeping to a healthy diet with lots of fresh food such as pineapple, apples, mushrooms and avocados can be beneficial to keeping joint pain under control.

Remedies to help with Joint Pain:

- Heat pads, warm baths or wheat scarfs are good for stiffness and can help with flexibility.

- Ice packs can help to numb the nerve endings dulling the pain down.
- Acupuncture can be good for balancing hormones and pain relief.
- Chiropractor or Osteopath can detect joints that are out of line.

Best Supplements for Joint Pain:

- Hormone replacement therapy (HRT)- this can be used to address joint pain and may be suggested by your GP, it is thought to relieve some of the symptoms of joint pain but not all.
- Calcium – good for bones during menopause which is important as Osteoporosis is a condition lots of women can get during the decline of Oestrogen which makes our bones more fragile and prone to breaking.
- Magnesium – is needed for calcium to be absorbed into the bloodstream, research shows that a magnesium deficiency can contribute to inflammation which leads to pain in the joints.
- Vitamin D – a lack of this can lead to weakness in the bones and joint pain. Sunlight is the best way to get Vitamin D, however in the winter months the sun is not strong enough, so a supplement is a good idea. Eating foods rich in Vitamin D is also recommended.
- Omega 3 – Lots of oily fish or taking a supplement would be the next best thing.
- Devils Claw – The root of this plant is commonly used to treat muscle and joint pain.

- Arnica- a well-known traditional remedy for relieving aches and pains and bruising.
- Glucosamine – a great supplement to start taking at the beginning of menopause as a preventative measure, it can help reduce deterioration of joint tissues which means you avoid joint pain later on! It can also help to prevent other joint conditions such as osteoarthritis.

Ladies, don't suffer in silence, there are lots of different remedies you can try to cure joint pain so be sure to book an appointment with your GP to rule out other conditions and get yourself some help!

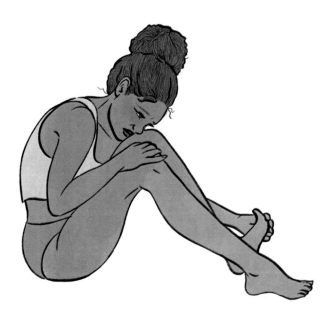

Vaginal Dryness (Atrophy) and Low Libido

Around 70% of women worldwide suffer with Vaginal Atrophy (thinning and drying of the vaginal walls that occurs when Oestrogen decreases), yet even more shocking is that less than 7%, yes 7% of women will receive treatment for it! The more I have researched this topic the more shocked I have found the whole conversation, or lack of conversation around this topic to be! Symptoms can include, soreness, itching, burning, urinary problems and some women have trouble sitting down. This can have some devastating effects on woman, from painful sex to low libido and not wanting sex at all, some women have told me it is the 'dreaded chore' and the bane of their lives that causes relationship issues with their partners who cannot understand what has changed. There IS so much help out there and you shouldn't be suffering in silence, go and speak to your GP and don't take no for an answer!

Symptoms:

Women who are Perimenopausal, Menopausal and post-Menopausal can suffer with Vaginal Atrophy, yet some women may never suffer with it at all. Symptoms include...

- Pain or burning when urinating.
- Spotting after intercourse.
- Pain during sex.

- Urinary incontinence.
- Thinning of the vagina walls.
- Vaginal burning.
- Vaginal dryness.

Causes:

Again, due to the decline in Oestrogen, the Vaginal tissues thin and dry out, also loosing elasticity. There are other times that this may happen including:

- Surgical Menopause when the ovaries are removed.
- Chemotherapy.
- During breastfeeding.

Regular sexual activity helps keeps the vaginal tissues healthy, another added benefit of a healthy sex life is the circulatory system and heart health benefit too.

Risk Factors:

Women who have never given birth naturally are more prone to vaginal atrophy, smoking can also affect blood circulation, depriving the vagina tissues of oxygen.

Possible Complications:

Vaginal Atrophy causes changes in the acidity of the vagina making it easier for yeast and bacteria to thrive. It can also increase the risk of urinary system atrophy, leading to urgent urination, more frequent visits to the toilet and a burning sensation when urinating.

Diagnosis:

Always see your GP with any of the above concerns, if intercourse is painful, even with lubrication. Any vaginal bleeding, discharge or burning should also be discussed with your GP. Some women are embarrassed to talk about intimate problems, but it is so important to seek medical advice to avoid any further complications. They may refer you to a Gynaecologist for tests and ask you lots of questions to diagnose vaginal atrophy. Your GP can also examine your genitalia for signs of Vaginal Atrophy, these signs can include:

- Pale, smooth Vaginal lining.
- No elasticity.
- Stretching of uterine support tissue.

Your GP may also carry out a vaginal smear test, acidity test and send you for a blood test.

Treatment:

Over the counter moisturisers and water-based lubricants can help with dryness. Your GP may recommend using an Oestestrogen replacement therapy which can be taken orally or topically.

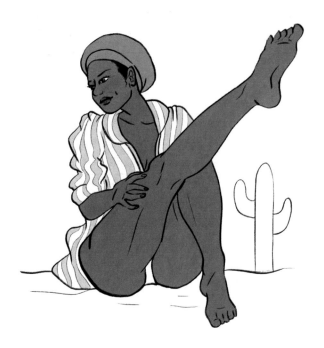

Prevention:

Wearing loose-fitting clothes and cotton underwear can help, staying sexually active helps with blood circulation in the vagina and stimulates moisture. Vitamin E oil can be used as a lubricant and Vitamin D increases moisture in the vagina.

Low Libido during Menopause

When you are going though Menopause, you will possibly notice that your sex drive (libido) is changing. Some women will notice an increase in libido, but most go through a libido decrease, it is very very common, this happens due a decrease in hormone levels. Often leading to vaginal dryness and causing pain during intercourse, this leads to a lack of interest in sex.

You can try to increase your sex drive with lifestyle changes or sex aids and lubricants, but if that does not work your GP can help you find the right treatment, so always speak to them for help and advice.

Menopause can affect libido in many ways, with your testosterone and Oesteogen levels decreasing it makes it difficult for you to get aroused. Vaginal Atrophy and dryness often cause discomfort during sex, leading to a lack of interest in intimacy.

Other factors like weight gain and other physical changes to your body during the menopause can affect your libido and decrease your enthusiasm for anything physical/sexual. Feeling tired due to lack of sleep, night sweats and irritability can also make you feel uninterested in sex. Another huge turn off from anything sexual is depression and anxiety.

See your GP:

Your GP can help determine any underlying causes of lack of libido during Menopause, and may advise treatment such as:

- Prescription Medication.
- Home remedies.
- Over the counter Medication.

Remember that our GP's talk about these issues more often than you think and their job is to look after your health and wellbeing. If it is a difficult conversation for you to have here are some ideas that might help:

- Write down all your worries, it will help your GP if it written down and you will not forget everything you wanted to say.
- Be honest with your answers.
- Ask for a female GP if its easier for you to be more open.

Treatment:

- HRT (Hormone Replacement Therapy) – This can work by helping reduce vagina dryness and replacing the hormones your body is no longer producing.
- Lubricants – There are lots of different lubricants on the market, they can help your libido and ease pain and discomfort during intercourse.
- Exercise: Great for keeping weight gain at bay and lifting your mood by releasing endorphins and reducing stress.

Communication:

Speak candidly to your partner and be honest about how you feel, remember you are in this together and if you are keeping the lines of communication open this might help with your mood and libido by talking about how you feel. It is not always about sex, sometimes just to be close to your partner makes them/you feel close.

If you are affected by any of the above, always go and speak to your GP, there are lots of different remedies and treatments they can recommend that are tailored for you and your symptoms.

"

Menopause is a biological reality that all women go through in many different ways, to different extremes & with hugely varying consequences.

We're all unique. There really is no need to suffer in silence anymore, we're entitled to the support we need to manage this time in our lives, regardless if that help is HRT, a more holistic approach, or both! Understanding is the first step, asking for help the second.

- Sharron Davies MBE

Weight Gain

This is a topic that always creates a huge stir amongst my friends, my Menopause group, and posts for clipboardclaire.com. With the average woman after the age of 40 gaining about 1 pound a year, the average weight gain is likely to increase even more with hormonal and physical changes which take place as we go through the Menopause.

Weight gain can often leave many women feeing low and self-conscious, especially if they have been active and fit and in good shape for most of their lives. For most women, the weight tends to sit around their middle and once there, it can be exceedingly difficult to lose. Lots of women try crash dieting and cannot understand why they cannot just eat sensibly for a few weeks, and the weight will come off, like they could do in their younger years. Lots of women notice weight gain during perimenopause which can be 10/12 years before the Menopause. There are lots of factors that play a role in weight gain around the Menopause.

Why do we gain this weight?

With hormones fluctuating as you enter the Menopause, (Oestrogen can elevate and decrease, both causing increased fat storage) this causes your body to deal with your food intake differently and often this results in weight gain. As we get older, our metabolism (the rate of calories you burn) begins to slow down and reduces, causing us to store more calories and not burn them off like we used to be able to do. Lack of exercise will make this even worse, so keep on exercising regularly and keep on moving. Going through the Menopause can be a stressful time and the hormone cortisol will increase, when this happens you are more likely to develop weight around your middle. Lots of women also suffer with poor sleep, or inadequate sleep, this has also been linked to weight gain.

What can we do about weight gain?

The most effective way to combat menopausal weight gain is to counteract it (prevent the weight from building up) eat less and exercise more. Its all about being in a calorie deficit to lose weight and maintain it. It has also been suggested that women burn less calories during and after the Menopause when they rest. Insufficient calorie intake and decreased muscle mass can increase your risk of osteoporosis too, so what you eat is going to have a huge impact on your weight going through this transition period in your life.

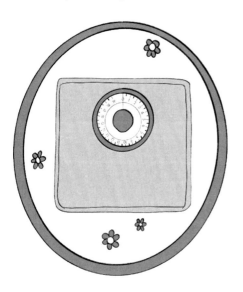

- Eat a healthy, well balanced diet that gives you all the nutrients you need. Make sure you have enough protein, vegetables, and fresh fruit. This will keep you at a healthy weight and help you in the long term, drastic dieting rarely works, and you put all the weight back on again, leaving you disheartened.
- Goli Gummies – Made of apple cider vinegar, these have been said to aid weight loss as well as many other health benefits.
- Keeping toned, especially your muscle at this time is key, as they are

more effective at burning calories than fat. Muscle mass decreases naturally and from that alone you will gain weight.

- Exercise – This is the most effective way to lose weight, but once or twice a week is not enough as we get older and go through this period of our lives. You need to be doing exercise most days in some way, shape or form. Aiming to do 10,000 steps a day is a great way to log your exercise. Whether it be walking, cycling, swimming or a yoga class or even housework and gardening, this all adds up to keeping in shape and keeping our excess weight off.
- Supplements – There is no tablet out there that can help you lose weight, but some have been linked to making you feel fuller and can aid weight loss along with a calorie-controlled diet.

- GP – If you are really struggling with weight gain see your GP, they can help you find a solution and suggest ideas that might motivate you and help you in the long run.

The Low Carb Diet

A Low carbohydrate diet is excellent for weight loss and helps reduce abdominal fat, you can still eat carbs and lose weight, but you do need to cut back on eating too many.

A Mediterranean Diet

Always been known for reducing heart disease and improving your health, a Mediterranean Diet can also help you to lose weight too.

Vegan/Vegetarian Diet

This can be another weight loss option but including milk and cheese has been shown to work well in older woman.

Other changes that can help with weight loss:

- Good quality sleep – lots of women have trouble sleeping during the Menopause but having a good night's sleep is important for maintaining weight. Women are more likely to be overweight who sleep badly or too little.
- Acupuncture – This may help increase Oestrogen levels which can help promote better sleep, leading to better weight management.
- Stress – Yoga can be great for reducing stress, if you are stressed, cortisol levels rise which can be associated with weight gain.
- Green Tea – Drinking green tea can help with burning fat.

If you want to lose weight, it is important that you put a plan in place for the long term, there are no quick fix overnight solutions. Regular exercise, eating the right foods, and getting a good night's sleep is the best way to lose and maintain a healthy weight as you go through your Menopause.

Sleep Issues

There is truly nothing worse than Insomnia! I have been there and "got the T- shirt"! I can quite honestly say, it was 7 months of hell and some! Trying to get anyone to actually believe that I had NO sleep whatsoever at night fell on deaf ears.

We are supposed to aim for about 7 hours sleep a night, and lack of it can have a huge detrimental effect on us. Our mental health can suffer, we can have heart problems, and our cognitive function goes out the window totally! As we go through the Menopause, our sleep plays a major part and can also influence other heath conditions at this time.

It is down to, again the decline of Oestrogen that can cause disrupted sleep. All of the following can cause you to wake up or not be able to get to sleep in the first place: Hot Flushes, Night Sweats, Anxiety, Depression. Some of these symptoms could actually be the cause of bad sleep, with Anxiety and Depression being caused because of the lack of sleep! Problems such as joint pain and constantly needed the toilet at night are also to blame for sleep disturbance, due to the decline in Oestrogen. Progesterone decline also plays a part in sleep disturbance as it has a sleep-inducing effect on the brain's pathways.

Some of my friends tell me they suffer horrendously with Restless Leg Syndrome, when I looked into this, it seems women are far more likely to get this than men. You get a tingling and creepy crawly sensation in your legs but only at nighttime. Post-Menopausal women suffer more than women who haven't started the Menopause. What is left unanswered is whether it contributes to poor sleep or women are more aware of it, because they are awake.

Some suggestions for poor sleep include: Stress management, healthy eating, exercise, being socially active.

Some other ideas that have been suggested to me to improve sleep are:

- Having a good bedtime routine. This is good for establishing a good sleep pattern.
- No afternoon snoozing!
- Do not exercise too near to going to bed.

Before bed:

- Have a soak in the bath to relax.
- Read a book, but nothing that will get you thinking about it afterwards!
- Do not eat too near to going to bed.

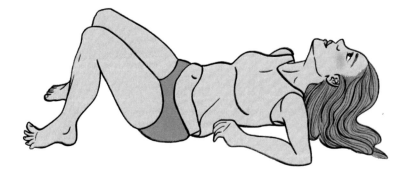

- Alcohol should be avoided if possible as it does not help you sleep.

Bedroom Set Up:

- Do not have the room too hot but not too cold either.
- Make sure the room is dark, and noise free.
- Make sure you have a good mattress and are comfy.
- Use good quality bedding.
- Avoid TV, Mobile Phones and working on a Laptop before going to sleep.

There are Herbal Remedies on the market too, which can aid better sleep, but I think its down to trial and error and what works for you. Some of these have been highly recommended by friends who are having trouble sleeping at night.

- Nytol Herbal,
- Super Sleep from Webber Naturals,
- Melatonin Supplements (This is the hormone that your body produces, telling your brain it is time to sleep),
- Magnesium (Can help to relax the mind),
- Lavender (Smelling this before you go to sleep can enhance your quality of sleep),
- Passionflower (Popular remedy for insomnia).

Always consult your GP, if you are concerned about an underlying sleep problem and especially if it goes on for months on end. If your daily life is being affected, do not suffer, there is help out there.

Why is fitness important during menopause?

Exercise isn't a proven way to reduce menopausal symptoms, however, regular exercise can help youmaintain a healthy weight, relieve stress and improve your quality of life, which is why I feel so passionateabout promoting it.

Exercise during and after menopause offers many benefits, including:

- Preventing weight gain- Due to hormonal changes & often lack of sleep, women will be prone to losemuscle mass and potentially gain abdominal fat during menopause. By introducing a regular exerciseroutine, especially one focused on strength training you can help maintain muscle mass and reduce fatgain.

- Increase bone density- Strength training increases bone density which is vital during and aftermenopause, as this lowers the risk of fractures and osteoporosis.

- Reducing the risk of other diseases- Menopause weight gain can have serious implications for yourhealth such as increasing the risk of heart disease and type 2 diabetes. Regular exercise can counterthese risks.

- Boosting your mood- The Menopause can take its toll on women's mood. Exercise has the oppositeeffect and in turn, helps lower the risk of depression and cognitive decline.

When choosing the type of exercise to partake in during the menopause, you may want to consider your exercise options and their benefits:

- Aerobic activity- Aerobic activity is easily accessible and endorphins often flow whilst doing it. Briskwalking, jogging, biking, swimming or aerobics are to name a few.

- Strength training- Around age 30, you begin losing roughly 1% of your muscle mass each year. Becausemuscle burns fat, this actually leads to fat-based weight gain. You can reverse this process and fightosteoporosis by weight training.

- Stretching/Yoga/Meditation- Stretching/Mindfulness and Yoga style activities can not only help reducestress and calm the mind but also improve flexibility.

Lynsey Suzanne Treharne - Founder of Fitness in 15 and Lynsey Suzanne Fitness

Anxiety

I look back now and realise that for me all the signs were there, but I convinced myself I was fine, when I blatantly was not! It is always a case of if only we knew then, what we know now. Personally, it could have saved me many years of suffering and I mean really suffering.

I guess we all kind of feel the gradual onset of the Menopause, but for some it is an extremely turbulent time. Where your hormone levels start to drop or like mine virtually bottom out overnight, leaving me, not only in agony with my joints, but playing havoc with my mental health too. We always think we are the only one, but with the endless Menopause groups I now belong to on social media, if there is one thing that is spoken about more than anything (even hot flushes!) it's Anxiety and for some Depression.

I have talked to lots of my friends over the years and now believe some of them could have been suffering the same and like me maybe not have known it. With the chemicals changing in our brain, this may affect in turn your mood. For me it was a gradual process and as I also had other things going on in my life that were also making me very unhappy, I put it down to that as opposed to anything to do with the Menopause.

With fluctuating Oestrogen and Progesterone levels, this can cause feelings of Anxiety or Depression, leading some women to develop Panic Disorder during the Menopause too. Some women could be more prone to Anxiety at this time if you suffered with Postpartum Depression and be more likely to suffer with Panic Disorder. These are not one-off Panic Attacks; these are regular and often brought on by worrying about when the next Panic Attack will strike. The symptoms can vary from one woman to another, some have heart palpitations and others become sweatier. Not easy to diagnose apparently but it can be treated by your GP who should be able to help you.

With constant changes in our hormones, this could be responsible for influencing the neurotransmitters in the brain, possibly being a cause of Depression at this time. If you start to struggle with work, home life, relationships, friendships and cannot see a way out, it is time to have a word with your GP. Definitely, if you have feelings of suicide, or are feeling increasingly negative about everything, have no one you feel you can confide in or are struggling to make sense of it all, see your GP or a good Therapist. They can often offer a helpful outsider's point of view

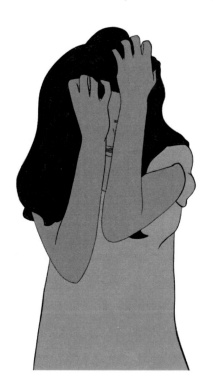

with the issues that are most important to you and troubling you. CBT (Cognitive Behavioural Therapy) can be helpful to some, this is a talking therapy, that can help you manage your problems by changing the way you think and behave. Others need more conventional methods, in the form of Anti-depressant tablets, they work by balancing the chemicals in the brain that effect your mood and emotions. They can also help with sleep, concentration, and relaxation, and can be for short term or long-term use. Again, speak to your GP, they will advise you which method is best for you and will help you through this time.

There are lots of ways to cope with emotion at this phase of our lives, a healthy lifestyle being the main one. Exercise is key and helped me greatly, going to the gym 4 or 5 times a week and releasing those endorphins helped to lift my mood and lots of my friends say they do the same. Meditation and Mindfulness (just having time on your own in silence, listening to the things around you and you breathing) has become very popular. Trying a new hobby or setting yourself realistic goals and having a sense of achievement, all aids in a positive and happy mind set. Speak to friends and family, make sure you connect with someone, do not shut yourself off at this time. Take Vitamins and Natural Products and make sure you get lots of fresh air and be with people who lift you up and not drag you down.

Take time for yourself and make sure you have things to look forward too, however small they are. Time out with a friend, a special lunch somewhere, a long walk with some fresh air, all these things aid your mind.

Having been unaware myself that I was menopausal, and consequently taking anti-depressants to help with what I thought was a nervous breakdown, I welcome all initiatives that will aid other women in understanding their own bodies.

This book is a fantastic resource and I hope that it helps women to become more aware of the symptoms and find the right support and treatment that will help them to cope with what can be a very difficult phase of their lives.

I am so proud to be a part of the Menopause Revolution and delighted to see that support, like this book, is finally making the subject something that we can all talk about.

Carolyn Harris
MP for Swansea East

Depression

Every Woman's experience through The Menopause is different and the majority of Woman have symptoms that negatively affect their lives, whether this is through their family relationships, personal lives or is work related. The main reason for this is the decreasing levels of the hormone Oestrogen, and the effect it has on different areas of the body during The Menopause. This can have a big impact on your brain and your emotions, which can last for many years, through Perimenopause to Post Menopause.

Low mood and feelings of Depression can be very common symptoms of The Menopause, including having low self-esteem, anxiety, panic attacks, irritability, poor concentration and no energy. Lots of these symptoms can be mistaken for Depression and many women are given anti-depressants wrongly for these symptoms. It seems pretty normal to feel angry and more irritable going through this stage in your life, from speaking to my friends. Often if you have had Postnatal Depression in the past you are more likely to suffer with these issues during The Menopause.

So, what are the differences, and what do we need to look out for:

- A Depressed Mood;

This is pretty normal, and a brief time of feeling blue or sad is commonly experienced and does not require any treatment. This is referred to as Dysphoria.

- Depression, as a symptom;

This is often due to a wide variety of medical or psychological problems, or it can be due to an intense reaction to life events, maybe divorce, death, losing a job etc. Usually relatively short term and not requiring medical intervention, but it can lead to Clinical Depression.

- Clinical Depression;

This is believed to be a result of a chemical imbalance in the brain and requires medical treatment.

- Our Mood and Hormones;

A few clinical Menopause trials have found none of the above types of Depression to be related to the menopause. Women no doubt suffer with mood swings and extreme highs and extreme lows during Perimenopause when their hormone levels are fluctuating during the transition to Menopause. If your sleep is affected, due to night sweats etc this would definitely have a huge impact on your mood.

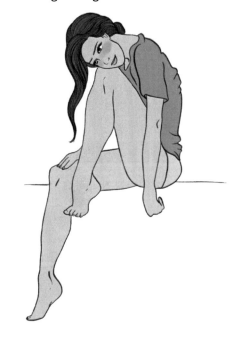

How can we deal with these feelings?

For mild symptoms, lots of my friends have taken St. John's Wort, a natural remedy and with some lifestyle changes, have felt a lot better. Also;

- Prioritise your life, set small goals for yourself, do what you can when you can.
- Exercise regularly, or do something you enjoy doing, and makes you happy, like going to the cinema or joining a new activity.
- Give yourself time, your mood might take a little longer to lift than you think.
- Don't make important decisions until your mood/depression has lifted. Talk things through with people that know you and will support you with your decision making.

Depression that is severe;

Always see your GP if you have suicidal thoughts and are drowning with life. Antidepressant medications can be taken to correct the chemical imbalance. Lots of women have a marked improvement taking these and with very few side effects, some have said it has made a huge difference to their Hot Flushes too. Counselling is another effective way to combat Depression and Psychotherapy can help too.

There is help out there, so please don't suffer in silence, talk to your friends and family about how you are feeling and know that you can get better in time.

So proud of all that you've achieved with this book- reaching out to so many and making it ok to talk about this subject.

Thank you for not only sharing your journey by going the extra mile to help others, including getting men and businesses talking about the menopause.

Dr Sarah Hazard

Brain Fog

For lots of women, this can be a very debilitating symptom of the Menopause. It can affect many aspects of your life, but especially your work and have a huge impact on your job. It has been reported that some 60% of women struggle to concentrate and remember things and this can start as soon as you hit Perimenopause It can also be linked to sleep issues, which is something I suffered terribly with for over seven months. I would go to bed and actually not sleep all night! When I say no sleep, I mean not half an hour's sleep! How I coped at that time, I will really never know, but I just did. It did get so bad that I visited my GP as it became so bad. I tried lots of relatively strong drugs, that she gave me but nothing worked and I just had to hope that it would stop, which it did.

Apparently, the brain fog is all to do with the hormone changes, Oestrogen and Progesterone which are responsible for doing different functions including cognition. I am forever forgetting what I have gone upstairs for and quite often my girls finish my sentences for me, of course, I have finished those sentences in my head long before, and I'm off doing the next thing on my list! I did think a few years ago maybe I had a mild case of Dementia or Alzheimer's! I think I have it relatively mildly compared to lots of women and I am told in time it should just go away on its own.

I am told a Mediterranean Diet may help with Brain fog as is often rich Omega-3 fatty acids. Foods that are good for brain fog include fresh fruit and vegetables, fish, olive oil, beans, and wholegrains and nuts.

I also think the Brain Fog may have played a big part in my insomnia a few years ago, sleep problems are high on the list for women going through the Menopause. I think most women at some stage will have some sort of sleep issues. I try not to eat too late, do not drink too much caffeine just before bed and try and relax before going to sleep.

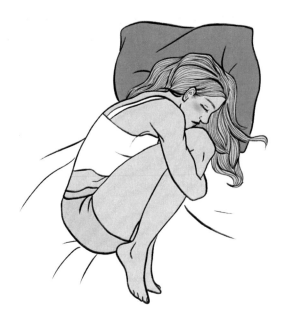

Again, Exercise is great with any memory problems, cardiovascular exercise as many times a week as you can manage, including walking, jogging, cycling, swimming and lots of strength training, can all aid memory issues.

I did laugh when I was told that my brain needed to work out, and doing crosswords or learning something new was great for keeping the brain active. Post It pads are my new best friend, and I write most things down on them, unlike my daughters, I don't use my phone to write things down as I often forget to look at what is on my list. I prefer it to be physically written down or there is no chance of me remembering it!

Lots of my friends that still work, often tell me they forget important things and make mistakes at work and it's very frustrating. I have some very robust friends and this can have a huge effect on your confidence and feel an inability to produce work to the high standard they could years ago. I think with the media and more people talking and covering the Menopause, employers are having to sit up and take notice, considering 50% of the population are female. I watched a programme not so long ago and it was actually the Police Federation that allowed the female staff that were suffering with the Menopause and its effects , to work from home and come in a bit later if it helped with their symptoms . I think this is a great idea and for some of my friends who suffer massively with this, believe it should be rolled out across the country, I think less sick time off would be had and companies would get much more from their workforce.

A Fabulous Menopause book! So refreshing to
read a book on this subject that
is easy to understand. I am sure many women
will benefit from this and many can relate.
Well done!
Being in premature menopause myself at just
age 13 this would have been such a good book
to read!
So hats off to you for getting this book out
there Claire!

- Natasha Owens
(@natashaowens4134)

Bloating

This is something I get asked about all the time! So, I decided to investigate Menopause Bloating a bit deeper to try and find some solutions and find out why it happens.

Often this starts during the Perimenopause stage (the beginning of the Menopause), causing your stomach area to feel over-full and often swollen. For some women it can cause pain and discomfort and make other parts of the body feel swollen and bloated too.

Why and What causes Bloating during Menopause:

- Fluctuating hormone levels can be responsible for bloating especially during your perimenopause years. Oestrogen levels can be higher at this time and this increase causes the body to hold/retain water, leading to bloating.
- A build-up of gas in your gastrointestinal system that can be caused by;
  Smoking
  Stress
  Diet
  Exercise

Post-Menopause bloating is more likely to be caused by the build-up of gas because your hormone levels have subsided and do not fluctuate like they did during Perimenopause and Menopause.

Solutions and treatments to prevent Bloating:

- Diet – Keep a diary of what food you eat and see if there is a particular food or group of foods that cause you to bloat. Often, fatty foods or processed food can cause bloating and even some vegetables can cause extra gas. Try to avoid foods with high levels of salt or sugar too.
- Exercise – The more exercise you do the less bloating will occur, that often means at least 5 times a week and varying what you do. Do lots of cardiovascular exercise one day and the next, swimming or yoga.
- Hydration – it is so important to stay hydrated to AVOID bloating, so drink lots of water through the day.
- Alcohol and Smoking – cause lots of bloating, so keep to a minimum if at all.
- Chewing gum – this can lead to filing your stomach up with air.
- Fizzy drinks – Carbonated drinks fill up your stomach with air, leaving you bloated.

If the symptoms are not improving, speak to your pharmacy, there are over the counter remedies you can try and if they do not work your GP can prescribe other medications that can prevent bloating.

- HRT – This can regulate your Oestrogen and Progesterone levels, helping with lots of menopause symptoms.

- Diuretics – Your GP would prescribe these to help your body avoid holding on to too much water.
- Probiotics - I highly recommend Probiotics and these are brilliant for bloating and gut health.

Weight Gain and not Bloating?

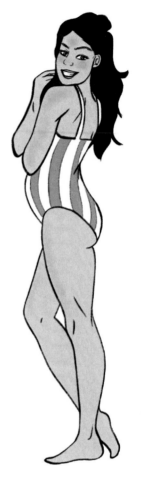

Going through the menopause can cause you to gain weight more quickly and mainly around your middle, in particular your stomach area. It can be hereditary and lifestyle, as well as ageing and not just the Menopause. Often Menopause bloating happens at the time of your menstrual cycle, eating large meals and quickly, can cause bloating too. This might make your stomach stick out and go down in size as the day goes on but it will not do this if it is weight gain. Weight gain is a common symptom of the menopause, but keeping your food portion sizes down, exercising regularly, getting enough sleep, and taking good care of yourself, should help with keeping any extra weight off.

Any prolonged and painful bloating should always be checked out with your GP, it can in rare cases be a sign of Ovarian Cancer or other health issues.

Most women suffer with bloating at some point during their journey through the menopause, but the good news is it should diminish after Menopause or subside considerably.

A brilliant book with clever tips to help soothe the inevitable ups and downs during the mid-point of a woman's life!

- Lucinda Miller
(Clinical Lead at NatureDoc)

Osteoporosis and Bone Issues

When we were younger and hitting the night clubs, knocking back the booze, smoking to be cool, it seemed to be the trendy thing to do. All these things will take a toll on your bones later in life, and especially going through the Menopause. Even if you did all these things then all is not lost you can still improve your bone health with a few lifestyle changes. From 40 years old our bone mass begins to decline; the body has been replacing old bone with new bone continuously up until about this age. This is definitely a time to look after your bones a little bit more! The Menopause without a doubt, effects your bone density due to a drop in Oestrogen, and could be up to as much as 20% bone density loss, 7 years after the Menopause.

It's all down to the basics we all know and should be adhering to at this time...

- Stop smoking: this can cause the onset of early Menopause, leaving less time for Oestrogen to protect our bones.
- Alcohol: I never realised post-Menopausal women who drink more than 6 units per day have a far greater bone loss than women who drank minimally.
- Exercise: It goes without saying, that regular exercise is a must to keep the weight down, and strengthen our bones, this will increase our bone size too.

- Sunlight: Apparently, we need to be outside far more than we are, having a cup of tea or coffee outside in the morning or going for a walk at lunchtime. These things will all aid our bones during this time.
- Gaining weight: making a conscious effort to eat sensibly and eating a well-balanced diet and not overindulging is a must as our bones are hit the hardest with weight gain the most.

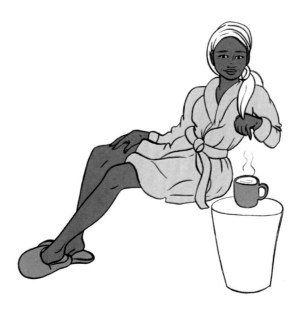

Foods that are great for stronger bones include:

- Green leafy vegetables such as Broccoli, Cabbage, Kale
- Fish such as Sardines and Pilchards
- Milk, Cheese, and any Calcium rich drinks
- Anything rich in Calcium and Vitamin D, it all helps.

I take some supplements that are high in Magnesium and Vitamin K too.

My GP has mentioned Osteoporosis (a health condition, making bones weak and more likely to break, often women don't know they have it until they break something and are tested, usually a bone density scan) to me a few times, possibly because of my horrendous joint problems, and again after a little research I try now to eat more apples, pears grapes and raisins. Zinc is another important supplement that can be worth looking into.

Obviously consult your doctor if you have any issues relating to this topic.

> None of us know when the menopause will start, how it will impact our lives or how long it will last. But it will happen and that's when advice and information from resources like this can really help. Claire is absolutely brilliant at the practical tips and tricks to help make the menopause easier, letting you know what is coming and how to manage it.

– Caroline Nokes
(MP for Romsey and Southampton North)

Irregular Periods

One of the main first signs of Menopause is usually a change in pattern of your periods. These can become very heavy or extremely light, and the frequency can be affected too. They may happen every few weeks or you may go months without one, until they stop altogether. Before your periods stop this time is called the Perimenopause (the first stage and takes anything up to 10 years for some women), and after 12 months of no period at all this is called Menopause and the stage after that is post Menopause.

When you have a period, the Oestgoen and Progesterone increase and decrease in a regular pattern. When Perimenopause begins your hormone levels are irregular and out of sync. This means you could experience irregular bleeding and spotting, and your period could be longer or heavier and the number of days between each one is different. You could also miss periods altogether but always consult your GP if this heavy bleeding occurs every few weeks or lasts longer than normal.

- Spotting

This is often light and between periods and is down to the changing hormones in your body building up the uterine lining or endometrium. This can occur before your period and as it finishes, and mid cycle can be common too.

Keeping a track of your cycle is key and tracking your periods can also help your GP diagnose what is going on quicker if they have the information in front of them. These can also help with many other

Menopause symptoms you may be suffering with but have not connected them to the Menopause.

- Abnormal Heavy Bleeding.

When your Oestrogen levels are high in comparison to your Progesterone levels, the uterine lining thickens, and this results in heavier bleeding as the lining sheds. Missing periods can also lead to heavier bleeding too. Heavy bleeding for a prolonged time can lead to Anaemia, so always consult your GP if it is affecting your daily life and you are having trouble with exercise or day to day life because of it.

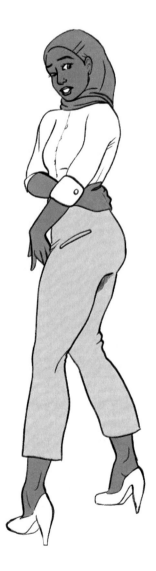

- Brown or Dark Blood.

The colour will often change from bright red to dark brown towards the end of your period, dark brown blood is a sign of old blood exiting the body. During Perimenopause you may see brown spotting throughout the month and notice the texture of blood may change and become more watery or thicker. If there is any odour this could be a sign of an infection, so always consult your GP.

- Shorter Periods.

With lowering Oestrogen levels, the lining of the uterine becomes thinner, hence bleeding may become lighter and shorter. This is often the case as you start Perimenopause.

- Longer Periods.

Towards the end of Perimenopause, your cycle may become longer and farther apart, normally 38 days or more are classed as longer cycles. These are often related to Anovulatory Cycles, which are cycles where you do not ovulate.

- Missed Periods.

With fluctuating hormones, you will no doubt miss periods altogether, sometimes not remembering when you last had a period at all. Once you reach a year with no period you have then reached Menopause. If you do still have periods now and again (this means you are still ovulating) remember you could still get pregnant!

- Managing Periods during the Perimenopause.

If you are suffering with cramps and pain and general discomfort, there are a few things you can try to help;

- Over the counter pain relief, or specifically designed period symptom tablets.
- Exercising to relieve the cramps/pain and bloating.

- Using a wheat bag or hot water bottle to the back or stomach to help with pain/discomfort.
- Try meditation or Yoga to help with relaxing and stress.

Always discuss any worries or symptoms that are a concern or not normal for you with your GP, these changes can be difficult and trying at times, but this is a new stage of your life and a time that offers new purpose and meaning.

Breast issues

Before and during the Menopause, it is very common to suffer with breast tenderness or pain. Mainly due to menstruation/periods and then as you transition through the Menopause, breast pain can return but from different causes. Sore breasts (also known as Mastalgia), are quite common during menstruation, this is down to hormonal changes causing fluid to build up in the breasts making them feel tender and sometimes swollen. During the Menopause, hormones fluctuate and are far more intense and dramatic, and can cause the breasts to become larger or smaller and change shape. It can often feel like a throbbing pain and sometimes feel like they are burning and a totally different sensation or experience to breast pain during menstruation/periods. After the Menopause, when your body stops producing Oestrogen, breast pain is much less likely and should subside, if not disappear completely.

Treatment for Breast Soreness/Pain:

As the Oestrogen levels start to drop as you go through the Menopause, breast pain and soreness should ease, but it can be worse going through the Perimenopause (beginning) stage.

- Take over the counter pain relief - Anti-inflammatory tablets can be good for breast pain.
- Reduce your salt intake – This can cause dehydration and worsen breast pain.
- Keep hydrated – Drinking more water aids hydration and can lessen pain.

- Avoid caffeine – This can help reduce breast tenderness.
- Bra support – Wear a more supportive bra and one that fits, it is worth having a fitting every year with all these changes going on.
- Warm/Cold compress – Apply a warm heat to your breast, this can help with pain. I am told these are amazing and worth buying!
- Hot bath/shower – Can help with pain/soreness.

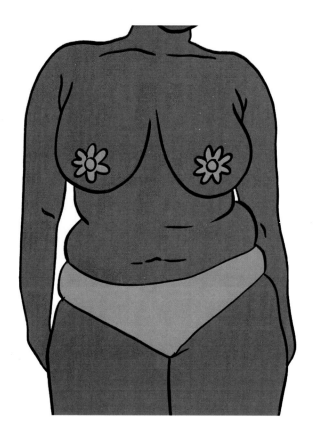

- Exercise – Gaining weight can cause breast pain too, so keeping active is important. A brisk walk daily can aid with keeping off those extra pounds.

See your GP:

Transitioning through the Menopause see's your breasts change in many ways, with cysts developing at the same time, many women worry about breast Cancer, but most of the time it is only normal changes to our bodies.

ALWAYS see your GP with any of the following, it may not be a Menopause issue and could be more sinister, and ALWAYS should be checked by your GP or Doctor, do not delay, for peace of mind get any of these issues checked out:

- Changes in texture to the skin.
- Swelling or lump under the armpit.
- Lump or firmness on the breast.
- Persistent breast pain.
- Increase in breast size.
- Clear, bloody or pus discharge from the nipple.
- Redness
- Change in appearance.

If you ever experience any chest pain, also seek medical help straight away as this could be a sign of a heart condition.

Keeping a note of breast pain is a good idea and then when you see your GP they can see when and how often the pain is occurring and helps them make a diagnosis.

Alternative treatments:

Natural remedies of good quality are often worth trying, as I have found out over the years. Popular supplements for breast pain/soreness include:

- Vitamin E
- Evening Primrose Oil
- Fish Oil
- Vitamin B

Sometimes just making a few lifestyle changes can give you relief from breast pain/soreness. Eating a healthy/ nutritious diet and not smoking or drinking too much alcohol or caffeine can help, and sometimes makes these symptoms far more bearable or disappear completely.

Bladder Issues

This affects lots more women than I ever imagined and the more I researched this topic the bigger the problem grew. Especially at the time of the Menopause, when women seem to suffer more than ever (even after childbirth), but worse still is that there are things you can do to stop or prevent urinary/stress incontinence and many women will not seek help for it, often because of embarrassment. Some women find that even when they laugh or sneeze, they might leak a small amount of urine, exercise or lifting heavy objects can cause leakage too. It can be a very minor loss of control but as we go into older age these symptoms can become worse. For some women you experience a sudden urge to go to the toilet and not be able to hold on until you get there.

What causes Menopause Stress/Urinary Incontinence?

During the Menopause when the Oestrogen levels are falling, you may notice that stress/urinary incontinence starts. This is down to the lack of Oestrogen causing your pelvic muscles to become weaker. You may no longer be able to control your bladder like you did before, and as you go through the Menopause the symptoms may become worse. There are different types that are associated with menopause, they include:

Stress Incontinence:

- This is the most common bladder control problem in older women. Weak muscles cannot hold the urine in when you cough, sneeze, laugh or exercise. This results in a small amount of leakage or can cause complete lack of control. This type of incontinence is usually caused by physical changes to the body, pregnancy, childbirth or menopause.

Urge Incontinence:

- This is when your bladder does not empty completely and can leave you with a constant urine flow or dribbling. Under activity of the bladder muscle can cause a weak urinary system and leave you with an increase in urinary hesitancy and needing to go to the toilet a lot at night (nocturia).

Other Issues that can cause bladder problems:

- Being Overweight – This can increase your risk of urinary incontinence because of the extra weight on your bladder.
- Medicines – These can have side effects attached to them which cause bladder issues if they have steroids or diuretics in them.
- Constipation – Long term straining with constipation can also cause your pelvic area to weaken.
- Infection – If you have a bladder infection or urinary tract infection, you may have temporary urinary issues, but these should improve when the infection has gone.

- Caffeine – This can make your bladder fill quicker, causing you to need the toilet more often.

What can you do to treat these issues?

Depending on what type of urinary incontinence you have and what is causing it, your GP may suggest some lifestyle changes to help, these may include;

- Losing weight - to take the pressure off your bladder and muscles
- Pelvic floor exercises - to strengthen your pelvic floor muscles.

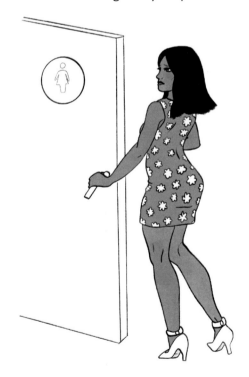

- Coffee – stop drinking as much or cut it out altogether to see if this helps.
- Nerve Stimulation – your pelvic muscles are electrically stimulated to help you regain control of your bladder.
- Medication – There are numerous medications that can help reduce symptoms, some calm the bladder if overactive, some increase the amount of urine your bladder can hold, and some Oestrogen products can help to tone your vaginal area.
- Surgery – this can lift your bladder into a better position and repair any damage to it.

Lots of Urinary/Stress Incontinence issues are temporary and will improve in time but some are more permanent. Always go and see your GP and do not be put off by the embarrassment, they can talk you through your options and plan. Millions of women suffer with these issues every day, and there are lots of different ways that this can be treated.

Fatigue and Dizzy Spells

I never realised there was such an issue as Menopause Fatigue but looking back I think there were times that I pushed on, even though I was on my knees with tiredness. I put this down to the lack of sleep and just life and my workload, but definitely looking into this has made me think I suffered with this.

Fatigue is a sure sign that you are beginning your journey through the menopause. As you go into Perimenopause, your hormone levels rise and fall, until your body stops producing them altogether. Whilst this is happening lots of other menopause symptoms will appear at the same time, hot flushes, anxiety, night sweats, irregular periods, weight gain etc, all of these can have a huge affect on your mood and energy levels, leading to fatigue. These symptoms can also leave you not sleeping at night and tired during the daytime.

What to do to combat Fatigue:

- Exercise – as much as it is the last thing you want to do, exercise actually helps, and studies have shown women who have a moderate to high intensity exercise regime actually have higher energy levels.
- Good sleep routine – going to bed at the same time and waking at the same time can help you establish a good sleep routine and leave you feeling more energetic. Having a good routine before

bed is equally important, maybe have a warm shower or bath before going to bed and avoid using anything with a screen so you are totally unwound before getting into bed.

- Keep cool – having your home too hot can also play havoc with your sleep pattern and leave you feeling too hot and overheated, especially if you suffer with hot flushes. Keeping your bedroom cool, keeps the body at a more natural temperature and aids sleep. Apparently 18°C is the perfect temperature.
- Do not eat too close to bedtime – Heavy meals too close to bedtime can leave you with heartburn and interrupt your sleep. Try eating smaller portions in the evening, and make sure your meals are healthy and nutritious.

There are lots of other factors that can lead to fatigue and are not necessarily down to the menopause, these other factors include:

- Alcohol
- Anaemia
- Depression
- Chronic fatigue syndrome
- Heart disease
- Lack of exercise
- Obesity
- Poor diet
- Stress
- Medications prescribed by your GP such as anti-depressants, pain killers, some heart medication and antihistamines.

If your fatigue is overwhelming you and having a huge impact on day-to-day life always speak to your GP, they will be able to talk to you about possible treatment options.

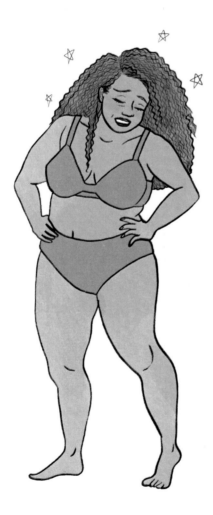

Menopause Dizzy Spells

Feeling woozy and lightheaded is apparently not uncommon during the Menopause, this is all down to the changing hormone levels affecting our circulation. Like many symptoms of menopause, it is not always clear why these dizzy spells happen, but with our Oestrogen and progesterone levels in decline, it is this that can have an effect on the blood vessels and circulation, resulting in dizziness as our blood pressure fluctuates. These declining hormones can also play a part in the functioning of our ears and heart too, also leading to us feeling off balance or dizzy.

Other symptoms of the menopause can cause us to feel like this too, including, hot flushes, panic attacks, and anxiety.

How to combat Dizzy Spells:

- Keep hydrated – with hormones fluctuating your body can struggle to retain water, and its super important to drink water to not get dehydrated.
- Anaemic - If you think you could be anaemic, ask your doctor to check your iron levels as this can lead to feeling dizzy if you have a low iron count.
- Ginger – this can help to stimulate circulation, so worth adding this to your diet.
- Eat at regular intervals – this will maintain your blood sugar levels and help maintain a steady supply of energy to the body.
- Stress – try keeping stress levels to a minimum, yoga, meditation and exercise can help combat this.

- List of foods – it is worth keeping a note of what foods you are eating and see if any trigger any dizzy spells for you.

See your Doctor or GP if you have any of the following, as it could be an underlying problem or issue that needs medical intervention.

- Feeling persistently lightheaded.
- Feeling like the ground is moving.
- Feeling like your surroundings are spinning.

As you go through menopause, most dizzy symptoms start to subside and go altogether. People are more likely to experience vertigo as they age, and women are more likely to get it than men. It could be that these dizzy spells are a sign of old age and not menopause after all, but more research is needed.

66

This is such a fantastic, informative & innovative idea - to actually provide help, support & reassurance for women going through the menopause & for younger women too - to help them look out for the common signs & how to help prepare for this stage of life. Such a super idea & proud to support it.

99

Daisy Harris- Reid
@mum_abouttown

Headaches

Lots of women find that the Menopause either fixes their hormone headaches or they get worse during Menopause. Most of us have had some sort of headache around the time of our periods a few times in our lives, so, what is the link and why do they get worse going through the Menopause?

There are 3 types of headache:

- Migraines – Most intense, pain increases on or both sides of the head and often pulsates and throbs.
- Tension – Often linked to stress, and not as severe as migraines, often feeling tightness or pain across the forehead and back of the head.
- Sinus – If your sinuses become inflamed, you often feel congested and can experience facial pain.

Menopause can affect your headaches in many ways, but like most things Menopause, each of us is different and we will experience different changes at different times. If you get hormone headaches usually, they might be less severe, or you may suffer less, or they may go completely. This is because your hormone levels stay low after your periods stop for good. Some women during Perimenopause have more frequent headaches and some who have never suffered before start getting them.

During Perimenopause migraines can become worse, often caused by the Oestrogen withdrawal and the decline of progesterone. Some women find that if they suffered with headaches due to their period they suffer more and have more severe headaches because of the inconsistency of Oestogen and Progesterone.

What can you do to treat these headaches:

- HRT (Hormone Replacement Therapy)

Your GP may suggest you try HRT for a number of Menopause symptoms, but this can be down to the individual and could make headaches/migraines worse or better. Some women have found that using Oestrogen skin patches work better than other forms of HRT when it comes to headaches.

- Change your diet:

Its worth keeping a diary of what you eat to see if any particular food triggers your headaches/migraines. When you next have a headache, write down what you ate a few hours before. The most common dietary triggers are, Alcohol, Cheese, Caffeine, Chocolate and Dairy.

- Exercise:

Regular exercise can help to prevent headaches, from a brisk walk to a high impact exercise class a few times a week. Always warm up slowly first, as getting straight into a workout could actually bring on a headache.

- Supplements:

Magnesium and Vitamin B-2 are good for preventing headaches, and Vitamin D is also beneficial.

- Acupuncture:

I have friends that say this has absolutely worked for them with headaches during the Menopause. This is a Chinese Medicine technique that uses needles to stimulate the body's energy pathways.

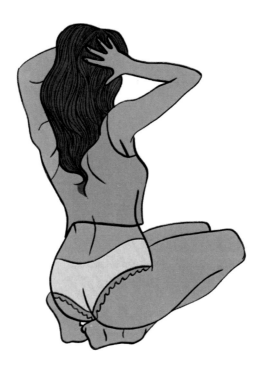

Lots of women say that the Menopause has stopped all their headaches, whereas some women say they suffer more than ever. They can be totally debilitating, with throbbing pain and the inability to look at light and being extremely sensitive to any noise.

Always go and see your GP with any symptoms that you are concerned about to rule out anything more sinister.

Mood Swings and Irritability

One minute you are happy, the next you are sad, then you really do not know how you feel! Its an emotional rollercoaster that you want to get off, but sadly, cannot. Some women feel like they are losing their mind or going mad, but rest assured you are not on your own!

Your mood can be affected by many different factors, from just waking up in a bad mood to having an argument with a loved one. It is not always obvious what causes these mood swings and the irritability that comes with them. Menopause seems to play havoc with our moods from Perimenopause through to post Menopause, causing us all to suffer. As your body starts to produce a lot less Oestrgoen and Progesterone in the lead up to the beginning of Menopause, your brain and body start to change too, altering your mood as well.

Causes of Mood Swings and Irritability:

Oestrogen helps to regulate lots of hormones, these may have mood enhancing properties, they can include;

- Dopamine
- Serotonin
- Norepinephrine

- Oestrogen supports certain brain functions and cognition is one of them, with lowering hormone levels this can lead some women to confusion and affects their mood in a negative way.

Lack of sleep is another big issue leading to mood swings, functioning on very little sleep is hard for anyone to do. Trying to cope with day-to-day life and a busy household and the normal 'ball juggling' that most women have to do, is even harder at this time and not surprisingly has a huge affect on your mood.

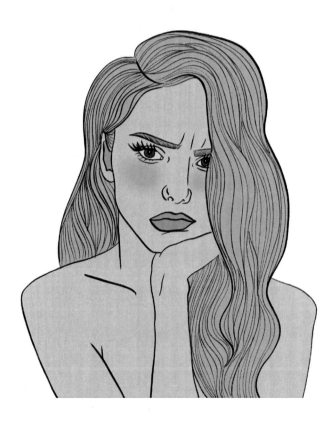

How to combat mood swings and irritability;

You may not be able to change your mood over night or completely, but these can help with mood swings.

- Exercise – Any type of exercise can help, anything that gets your heart rate up and those endorphins released will help with a low mood. Try to exercise regularly and keep to it, it releases lots of feel good chemicals into the brain. Sometimes a brisk walk is all it takes to make you feel better and picking a time to exercise that works for you, some like the mornings, others the evenings or after work. Listening to music or a podcast or audible book can take your mind off anything else on your mind.

- Healthy Food – this is vital to your mood and plays a bigger role than most women think. Eating a varied diet which contains lots of lean protein, fruit, vegetables and grains is likely to provide you with plenty of Omega-3 fatty acids and other nutrients that can improve your mood.

- Stress – Most of us suffer with it, it is impossible to avoid, but de-stressing can have a huge impact on your mood. Yoga, a quiet book read, or a relaxing bath can all help with a low mood and leave you feeling a lot better.

- Sleep – A huge mood changer is lack of sleep, not getting enough is a bad start to any day and your mood swings and irritability will be at its worst. Turning off all electrical gadgets an hour before

bed, making sure your bedroom is cool and avoiding caffeine and alcohol can help with getting a good nights sleep.
- Natural supplements – these can be a game changer for some women, always make sure they are a quality supplement for maximum effect.

- See Your Doctor;

Always see your GP or seek medical advice if your mood swings are excessive and you feel overwhelmed, they can help if your mood swings are:

- Causing Anxiety and Panic Attacks
- Making you want to avoid situations, people etc.
- Taking over your life

Always keep an eye on when and how you feel, Menopause Symptom Trackers are great for this, and will help your GP to diagnose you quicker.

- HRT (Hormone Replacement Therapy)

This can be used short term or long term for lots of Menopause symptoms but can be very good for alleviating mood swings and irritability.

- Acupuncture

This can help balance hormone levels and increases the production of dopamine and norepinephrine.

Mood swings and irritability tend to be more prevalent in Perimenopause and during Menopause, with some slight lifestyle changes your mood can improve dramatically. Once the hormone system stabilises, these mood swings should diminish.

Nausea and Digestive Issues

I never realised until I started researching and looking into digestive issues that gut health was so important during the Menopause and that it could have such a huge link to digestive issues. With our fluctuating hormone levels during perimenopause and declining levels of Oestrogen and Progesterone as we go through this transition time, there is no doubt in my mind that the gut is disrupted, and digestive problems set in!

Before the Menopause I could eat what I wanted and pretty much never had a problem with what I ate or drank. Fast forward to my Perimenopause, Menopause and now Post Menopause years and it was/is a whole different game! Personally, I never gave a thought to any stomach issues with the Menopause, we all think about hot flushes, bad sleep, irregular periods etc but now, I look at it all with a totally different perspective.

Morning Sickness/Nausea:

When going through Perimenopause, hormones are beginning to change, this can include changes to the FSH (Follicle Stimulating Hormone) which basically regulates ovary function. It works similarly to the early stages of pregnancy, hence the association to morning sickness. Lots of women say they wake up in the morning feeling nauseous when they are approaching the Menopause and have the feeling they might have had when they were first pregnant.

Declining Oestrogen levels can also cause Cortisol (the body's main stress hormone) to increase, raising blood pressure and reducing acid in our stomach, the result of which we end up with a poorly and upset stomach.

What can we do to avoid/stop this?

- Wake up earlier – Setting an alarm 30 minutes earlier giving your hormone levels extra time to settle as opposed to jumping up out of bed and rushing into your morning routine, should leave your stomach feeling much better.
- Eat breakfast – This is vital and will get those perimenopause digestive issues under control; a balanced healthy breakfast will stabilize your blood sugar levels and give you fuel for the day to keep you going and keep the nausea at bay.
- Chew properly – If you chew your food slowly and thoroughly, this will allow the food to be digested properly and make the body work less hard trying to digest it.
- Keep hydrated - Drinking water whilst eating your breakfast will help with nutrient transportation.
- Hate breakfast? – If like me, you cannot eat as soon as you get up, a smoothie is a good alternative breakfast to have.

Menopause Digestive Issues:

Oestrogen stimulates the muscle that lines the intestine, Progesterone has a relaxing effect on it, and they work hand in hand together. But during the Menopause, this is thrown out of its perfect pattern and is disrupted, resulting in, bloating, wind, indigestion, constipation, and diarrhoea. With Oestrogen dropping, the gut can be disrupted and can affect our food and waste products, leaving us bloated, having constipation or diarrhoea and for some Menopausal women, water retention and bloating which go hand in hand and are a persistent problem.

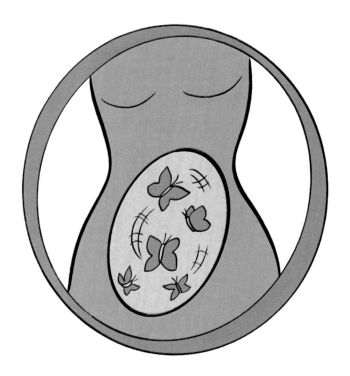

Menopausal Stomach Issues, Anxiety and Stress:

When our Cortisol runs low during the Menopause, blood pressure rises and our digestion slows down. Without Oestrogen's calming effect, adrenaline rises which in turn switches off our digestive function. This leaves us with sluggish bowels, stomach pains, cramps, bloating and constipation. If you suffer with anxiety during the Menopause (it is a very common symptom of the menopause) it is very easy to become flustered and stressed and feel you are not coping in stressful situations, this can cause tension and leave your stomach in knots.

I never realised the link to the brain and gut, so if you have a Menopausal upset stomach, it is worth checking out those tension levels, down to those pesky hormones again! The link between our mind and stomach means that any stress/anxiety issues we have, are going to be mirrored in our stomachs, and the muscles in the gut then becoming tense.

Menopausal Upset Stomach?

Along our intestine, there is a multitude of bacteria activity, and this is known as the Microbiome. Our Microbiome needs the right type of friendly bacteria to support our gut function and maintain our bowel movements. This plays an important role in keeping a Menopausal upset stomach at bay. These friendly bacteria produce vitamin B which is absorbed into our body, and this contributes to a normal energy metabolism, required for all our body functions and activities, particularly exercise.

What can we do to help with these Stomach Issues?

HRT (Hormone Replacement Therapy) – can provide relief from Menopause stomach issues.

Eat healthily – Phytoestrogens (Plant Compounds) mimic the effects of Oestrogen and can help balance hormones and help with digestive issues. These include:

- Legumes - Chickpeas, lentils and beans.
- Nuts – Almonds, cashews and peanuts.
- Seeds – Sesame, sunflower, pumpkin.
- Whole grains – rye, barley, oats, bran, granola, muesli, whole wheat.
- Soya Products – Yogurts, milk, flour, beans.
- Fiber – Broccoli, spinach, apples, cauliflower, whole grains.
- Omega-3 – Walnuts, egg yolks, salmon, mackerel, sardines, pilchards.
- Spices – Turmeric, great as an anti-inflammatory and can sooth and protect the stomach from acid.
- Fennel, cardamom, and caraway can also help with digestive issues. Great for combating wind and bloating.
- Sit down and eat – Eating on the go is not good for your digestion, sit down and chew your food and enjoy it!
- Do not chew gum – This can cause air to move in the wrong direction, causing you to burp.
- Peppermint tea - Drinking peppermint, chamomile and ginger tea can help with nausea and soothe your digestive system.
- Water – Good hydration is so important with digestive issues, and water will dilute acids that cause indigestion.

Supplements that may help with Digestive Issues:

- Evening Primrose Oil
- Peppermint
- Turmeric
- Omega-3

Probiotics can also aid digestion and help support your body's natural gut bacteria.

Always check with your GP before taking supplements as they can interfere with medication.

Electric Shock Sensations (ESS)

There are some pretty strange symptoms during the transition through the Menopause this one is no exception! I have lots of friends that would never have linked these to Menopause (or believed me that these are Menopause related) but after researching this topic for a long time now, they link these painful and sometimes debilitating symptoms to the Menopause!

My friends that have suffered with Electric Shock Sensations (ESS) explain them as a short, sharp shock of electricity going through the body at breakneck speed, leaving them in pain and/or very uncomfortable. I have been told it feels like a rubber band being snapped on your skin (ouch)! These are usually harmless and short-lived, but for lots of women, they experience these before having a hot flush.

What causes Electric Shocks during Menopause?

These sudden electric shocks come from the neurons in the brain that are misfiring, causing the pain you feel all over. No one seems to know exactly why this happens during the Menopause, but it is known that Oestrogen has an important role to play in your brain. With hormonal imbalances, the nervous system can misunderstand messages and lead to the neurons misfiring, causing these electric shocks. There are some medicines and medication that can contribute to ESS, and anxiety may increase the likelihood of having these electric shocks too.

What can you do about them?

As this symptom is related to hormones and sometimes anxiety can trigger them, you need to address those issues first to see if your symptoms improve or go away altogether.

- HRT (Hormone Replacement Therapy) – If your life is being disrupted by these electric shocks, it is always worth speaking to your GP about HRT, this can help with leveling out your hormones and minimize lots of unwanted menopause symptoms.
- Relax and unwind – Whether it is yoga, relaxing in the bath, meditation, walking, all these things will reduce your stress levels and anxiety, and help alleviate ESS.
- Phytoestrogens – this compound found naturally in soybeans, tofu, chickpeas, flax seeds, berries and green tea, all act like Oestrogen and level out some of the hormone dips.
- Vitamin B12 – Low levels in the body of Vitamin B12 can cause electric shocks, so see your GP, to have this checked.

Other Solutions to Help with ESS:

- Caffeine – This stimulates your nervous system which can contribute to ESS, so try cutting down or stopping altogether to see if your symptoms improve.
- Sleep – Sleep deprivation can affect all the body's systems and can exacerbate ESS.
- Alcohol and Smoking – These can both lead to nerve damage and actually cause ESS, so giving up, may stop these electric shocks happening totally.
- Hydration – Keeping your hydration up will help with all the systems in the body and overall, it will perform better.
- Exercise – This will always lift your mood and it reduces stress and anxiety which in turn can alleviate ESS.
- Healthy Eating – Your body needs the right nutrients to function properly, a diet rich in Omega-3, plant oils, and magnesium, all help with the function of the immune system.
- Supplements that may help with Electric Shock Sensations:
- Vitamin B12
- Omega-3
- Magnesium

Always seek medical advice from your GP with any new complaint as it could be more serious than you think and not linked to the Menopause. They can rule out anything more serious or any other underlying health issue.

"Exercise can provide multiple benefits through menopause, to feel strong, mobile, active, and energetic it's key to include strengthening, stretching, balance, and aerobic exercises into your life.

Aim for two resistance workouts per week to strengthen the body and include aerobic (cardio) exercise by doing 150 minutes of moderate-intensity exercise or 75 minutes of vigorous physical activity (VPA), or a combination of both.

-Michael Brigo
(@brigopt)"

Allergies

There are some bizarre symptoms that happen when we go into the Menopause, including allergies to things we never suffered with before. Just when we thought we had had enough thrown at us, we start coughing for no reason and sneeze at everything in sight!

Why do we start to suffer with allergies now?

It is all down to our Oestrogen levels declining as we go through the Menopause, and the impact it has on our immune system, making it react very differently to allergens. Whilst some women are already suffering with hot flushes, joint pain, sleep issues, digestive problems and so on, this puts a huge pressure on our nervous system. The body then starts to defend itself by producing more histamine (a chemical that leads to allergy symptoms). Dust, pollen, animals, and cleaning products now start to cause you to sneeze, cough and your nose to run as your immune system releases histamine to try to combat these issues.

Histamine and Hormones:

Some of us always start to dread the summer months in the back of our minds, as it is the season for hayfever! Having suffered as a child, then I did not suffer for years and now I get the occasional itchy eye and sneeze post menopause. For some women who have never suffered with hayfever, this can be another symptom that rears its ugly head.

Histamine is the body's chemical that is released when there is something irritating the body but can play havoc during the menopause too. It is a vital part of our immune system and normally works well and works hard to repair us, for example if you cut your arm and it starts to become hot, and even swollen, your immune system takes immediate action by releasing histamine.

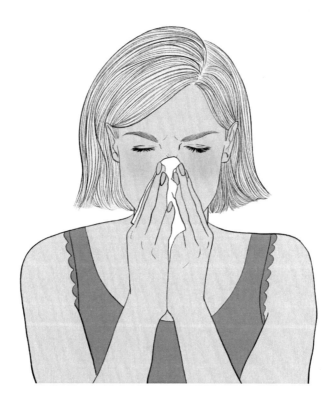

It opens blood vessels and allows more blood to get to the injured arm and the white blood cells fight off any possible infection.

But, during menopause we have so many other factors causing stress to our immune system that it causes the histamine to totally overreact, causing a lot of other menopausal symptoms by doing this. Menopause causes lots of problems with our immune system and there are a few reasons why:

- Stress to our Nervous System – Menopause causes stress to the nervous system, causing it to overfire, possibly having an effect on our immune system in turn.
- Tiredness – With hormones depleting, this makes us tired, and fatigue sets in, effecting our immune system.
- Sleep – With hot flushes and disturbed sleep, and possibly anxiety, this can have a huge effect on our sleep pattern, again effecting our immune system.
- Dehydration – A huge factor on our immune system is dehydration, this can lead to issues with our liver function, causing it to be stressed. The role the liver plays can have a huge part in deactivating histamine.

Allergies and Remedies:

- Asthma:

If you suffer with asthma, this may get worse as you go through the Menopause. Some women will develop asthma for the first time. Always see your GP with any breathing or wheezing.

- Food:

Becoming sensitive to certain foods you never had a problem with before, may mean you have an allergy to them, or that group of foods. Keep a diary and speak to your GP if the symptoms are worrying you.

- Eczema:

Our skin becomes much drier going through the Menopause and this may trigger Eczema. Your skin can become itchier and redder and inflamed and start to bleed. You can buy some over the counter creams for this, or your GP can give you a prescription for something stronger if it persists.

- Hives:

Menopause can be a super stressful time, and this can trigger lots of skin issues including itchy lumps or hives (nettle rash). It is a good idea to take an antihistamine tablet.

- HRT (Hormone Replacement Therapy):

HRT can work on lots of symptoms of the Menopause including allergies, and hives. Speaking to your GP about your options is a good idea, if the symptoms become unbearable.

Natural Products that may help:

Be careful when choosing washing powders and anything that is going on or next to the skin. Try more natural products. Lots of women say that Coconut Oil is an absolute game changer and great for dry skin.

- Vitamin C – A natural antihistamine and great if taken regularly.
- Probiotics – These can help with hay-fever and help with your immune system too.
- Vitamin E – May reduce inflammation when applied onto the skin.
- Magnesium – This helps to fight stress and aid the immune system.
- Calcium – Helps to reduce histamine production.

Menopause allergies often improve, if not go altogether, making some lifestyle changes and adjusting your diet can help with symptoms too.

Menopause is finally being talked about: on the radio, on TV, in newspapers and around the water cooler in offices. More women are going to their GPs about it than ever before but more still needs to be done to turn this natural life phase into a normal, non-taboo topic.

While the celebrities of this world seemingly leading the charge when it comes to menopause reform and discussion, there is a swathe of down-to-earth, everyday women behind the scenes, keeping this topic at the forefront of our minds. One such woman is Claire Hattrick, a formidable lady with whom I connected on Clubhouse this year and whose dedication to this topic so impresses me.
Claire's aim is to spread the word as far and wide as possible about menopause and its effects. Having suffered a number of symptoms herself, including terrible insomnia, she wants to forewarn and forearm younger women about what is, or could be, to come, and to help them better prepare themselves for the transition by making healthier life choices today.

This book is easy to read, practical and packed with information about pretty much every single menopause topic. Claire has done most of this work single-handedly, compiling this helpful book without the aid of a large publisher and for that I commend her. I truly hope her wish comes true and that this book gets into the hands of as many women in their 30 and 40s as possible.

-Katy Sunnassee (The Health Editor, Editorial Director of top santé magazine UK).

Burning, Dry Mouth and Dental Issues

Lots of my friends have complained that since starting or going through the Menopause they have had lots of mouth issues, so, I decided to investigate it. A burning mouth and tongue, gum problems, aching jaw and teeth are just some of the issues that women face at this transitioning time.

What causes Mouth Issues during Menopause?

With the levels of Oestrogen starting to decline during Menopause, this hormone is the one that is responsible for regulating the levels of fluid in the body. Falling Oestrogen levels can cause the mucus membranes in the mouth and nose to thin and become drier, this can affect the amount of saliva being produced. This can, in turn cause lots of mouth/teeth/jaw and gum issues, many of which can be uncomfortable and lead to problems with thirst, chewing and swallowing and effect your oral health.

Burning Mouth/Tongue: This can actually make you feel like your mouth is burning and on fire most of the time, but often it is a symptom that comes and goes. It is often caused by diet and your nutritional needs being a lot higher at the time of Menopause. Stress can be a big factor as well as anxiety, so if the symptoms worsen when you are stressed you know that you need to address the stress levels in your life. Anaemia is another thing to look out for, especially if you are suffering with heavy periods, your iron levels could be low. It is worth ruling this out by a blood test with your GP. Thyroid issues can also be connected to a burning mouth or tongue, if you feel you are continuously tired, have a low mood and maybe sleep problems too, its worth having it checked out with your GP.

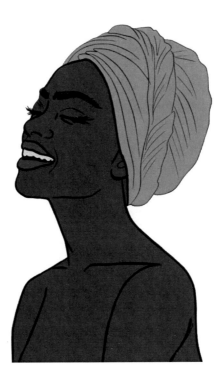

How to combat Burning Mouth/Tongue:

- Try using a good quality Multi Vitamin.
- Change your toothpaste.
- Change your mouth wash or any other mouth health products you use
- Try Alpha-lipoic Acid, this can work wonders for some women.

Gum Problems:

Lots of women seem to find that they start to get problems with their teeth and gums during Menopause. When brushing your teeth, the gums can bleed, and teeth become overly sensitive. It is always worth seeing your dentist and combating any problems before they become worse if they are causing you an issue. Women can also get sore teeth and a sore jaw, checking what hygiene products you are using and changing them to see if this makes a difference is definitely worth a try.

How to combat Gum/Teeth Problems:

- Try using a natural toothpaste for gums and teeth issues.
- Good quality Calcium and Magnesium supplements can keep your teeth healthy too.

Dry Mouth:

Menopause can also cause a symptom called 'Menopause Dry Mouth', it can cause your mouth, lips, and throat to feel sore, also leaving you feeling thirsty and maybe a little hoarse when you speak. Keeping your mouth moist can help, your saliva also helps to keep your teeth protected against decay and infections. Any changes to your saliva can give you a bitter taste and cause problems with chewing, tasting and swallowing and can lead to bad breath.

How to combat a Dry Mouth:

- Eating plain foods and fruit can help, avoiding hot, spicy and salty foods, as these dehydrate your mouth.
- Sucking hard boiled sweets and chewing sugar free gum, can increase the saliva in your mouth and even ice cubes can do the same.
- Avoid sugary, acidic foods as they can increase tooth decay.
- Apply a soothing lip balm, to avoid your lips from peeling and flaking and getting chapped.
- Take Sea Buckthorn Oil which contains Omega-7 oils, it is also great for supporting healthy mucous membrane.

Hair Loss, Brittle Nails and Body Odour

The strangest of symptoms can happen during the Menopause, some you can treat and find remedies for and others you cannot. Some of the symptoms can show as we get older anyway but can be exacerbated and made worse by the Menopause.

Hair Loss:

Due to lowered Oestrogen and Progesterone levels, hair loss can be quite significant. Both of these hormones help our hair to grow faster and stay on our scalp/head for much longer. Hair can become much thinner and grow much slower with declining hormone levels. Hair may also start to fall out in clumps when brushing your hair and can lead to bald patches, having a massive effect on a woman's self-esteem which is understandably upsetting.

Treatment:

- Speaking to your GP as early as possible after noticing the hair loss is vital. This will help determine the cause, it may be a nutrient deficiency and can be easily sorted out with a supplement.
- Your GP may do a blood test to check your thyroid and iron levels, again these can be sorted with medication.

- HRT (Hormone Replacement Therapy) can be an option, especially if there are other menopause symptoms it could help treat as well.
- Avoid stressful situations, if possible, this can play a huge part in hair loss with anxiety and depression, so keep your stress levels at a minimum.
- Exercise is great for a healthy lifestyle and makes you feel happier and stronger, this helps with a good hormonal balance promoting hair growth.
- Healthy eating and having a well-balanced diet are great for preventing hair loss.
- Drink green tea and take Vitamin B6 and Folic Acid supplements, these are are good for hair growth.
- Drink plenty of water and keep hydrated
- Avoid using heat tools, hair dryers, straighteners and curling rods etc as these cause breakages and make the hair weaker also causing it to dry out.

Always see your GP if you are losing hair in an unusual pattern, or rapidly and have any pain or other scalp issues.

Brittle Nails:

During Menopause, many women find that their nails become drier and more brittle, this is again down to hormone changes. They can also become flaky and prone to splitting and chipping. Oestrogen helps regulate fluid levels in the body and imbalances in Oestrogen

result in dehydration, weakening your nail's protective layer
of Keratin, leading to brittle nails.

Treatment:

- Eat a balanced diet, a lack of nutrients including Vitamin B, Calcium, and Folic Acid can contribute to dryness, splitting and flaky nails.

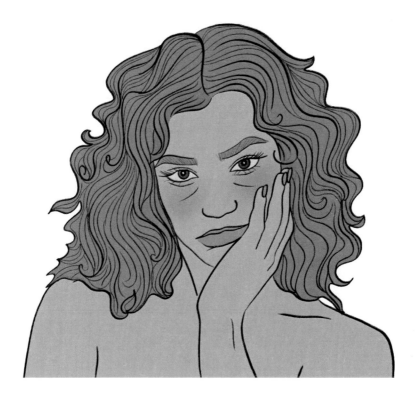

- Include plenty of protein, fatty acids, Omega-3, and Vitamin C in your diet too.
- Taking a nail supplement, can help protect your nails and make sure you have all the nutrients you need.
- Make sure your nails are kept well moisturised by using a good quality hand cream. Especially after showering or washing your hands to avoid them drying out.
- Wear gloves when you are doing chores.
- Keep your nails well-manicured, short nails can also help reduce the risk of breaks and splitting.

Body Odour:

Hormone imbalances and body odour go hand in hand, Oestrogen levels lowering can trigger hot flushes and night sweats meaning you sweat more which turns into more odour. With high levels of stress and often anxiety at this time, this can make you sweat too. Sweat itself is odourless but combine it with bacteria on your skin and it starts to smell. Anxiety sweat is produced by the apocrine glands, which are found under your armpits and groin areas, bacteria love these sweaty areas. When stress, anxiety and hormones settle down the body odour will do too.

Treatment:

- Cleansing wipes are great to carry around and you can freshen up anytime. Use one that is pH balanced and is as natural as possible.
- Zinc and Magnesium supplements can help other body odour too.
- Fabrics that allow your skin to breath i.e. cotton, wool and silk are great for keeping you cool and sweat free.
- De-stress as much as you can to avoid sweating, yoga and walking are great ways to ease stress and unwind.
- Avoid red meat, spicy food, garlic, and sugary foods as they can release compounds through the skin that contribute to odour.
- Drink plenty of water to keep hydrated, if you do not drink enough then you are likely to sweat even more.
- Natural deodorants can work wonders and keep unpleasant smells away, but still allow you to sweat naturally.

See your GP if the odour is starting to impact badly on your life, they can prescribe prescription strength deodorants and Botox to paralyze sweat glands. They will also check for other issues, such as your thyroid.

Menopause will directly affect
approximately half of the population.
It will indirectly affect the other half
too, whether as a partner, family
member, friend or colleague.

Too many continue to suffer due to a
lack of menopause information,
education, care and support.

We must be the generation to
#MakeMenopauseMatter

- Diane Danzebrink
Menopause Counsellor and founder of
Menopause Support and the national
#MakeMenopauseMatter campaign.

Muscle Tightness

Going through the Menopause I did have this symptom but put it down to the gym or my ongoing joint issues, but the more I have researched it, the more familiar the symptoms are to me! This is a more common issue with the Menopause than I first thought, as well as getting older, muscle tension can be linked to stress and anxiety during Menopause. Muscle tension is the feeling that the muscles are always tight and can be quite painful and an ongoing persistent problem. Cramps can also be a sign of muscle tightness too and happen to any part of the body.

What causes Tight Muscles during the Menopause?

With Oestrogen and Progesterone fluctuating, it is the hormonal imbalance that is the main cause of tight muscles. Both of these hormones play a part in causing this condition, low Oestrogen causes the levels of Cortisol to rise, raising blood pressure and blood sugar levels. The high level of cortisol and low level of Oestrogen cause the muscle to tighten in the body. Progesterone has a calming effect on the body and mind, but when the levels begin to drop due to menopause, the muscles become tense.

The muscles most commonly affected by this are:

Back, shoulders, and neck which in some cases can led to tension headaches. Mainly in the upper part of the body, but it can be all over that hurts at times. For some women it can lead to a bad and restless night's sleep.

Other factors that can cause Tight Muscles:

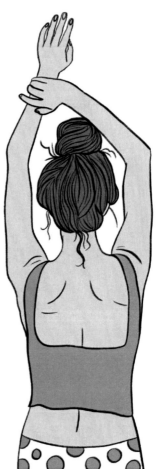

- Anxiety
- Stress
- Lack of Exercise
- Bad posture

What can you do for Tight Muscles?

It is mainly lifestyle changes that will combat Muscle Tightness, but there are some supplements that can help too.

- Stretching- Gently stretching your muscles can help ease the stiffness and pain.

- Magnesium – If you have low levels of magnesium in your body it can cause muscle cramps. Taking a good quality supplement can help and making sure your diet is rich in magnesium too.
- Exercise – Gentle but regular exercise is crucial for lessening muscle pain and can loosen the tension and pain. Walking, swimming, and cycling are great to reduce the effects of this symptom too.
- Diet – As well as magnesium rich foods, eating an iron rich well balanced diet and nutrient rich diet will relieve stress and muscle tension.
- Heat – A hot/warm shower or soak in the bath is great for soothing muscles, and a heat pack applied to the muscle can relieve pain.
- Posture – Lots of people don't think about their posture and the long-term effects and pressure it puts on their joints and muscles. It can affect any group of muscles but tends to be the back, neck, shoulders and hips.
- Deep tissue massage – This can help your body's circulation and soothe muscle tightness to help with relaxation and reduce your stress levels.

Herbal and Conventional Medicines:

You can buy over the counter pain relievers such as Paracetamol and Anti-inflammatory tablets for short term use, but if the problem persists you should see your GP. They may be able to offer alternative medication you can take and ensure it does not interfere with anything else you are currently taking. Herbal remedies may help as the muscle pain is down to hormonal imbalances, Soya Isoflavones can be great for naturally balancing Oestrogen, and another good natural supplement is Vitamin D, as it can aid muscle tension.

There are lots of different ways to relieve Muscle Tightness, always speak to your GP if you are struggling to resolve this at home or go to your local pharmacy.

Tinnitus

I post on a lot of Facebook groups and I hear them talk about Tinnitus and how it is linked to the Menopause, so thought I would do some research into it with the help of some friends who suffer terribly with it.

What is it and why have I got it now?

Tinnitus is an internal, often continuous (but can be occasional) ringing in one or both ears, it seems that the "pitch" can vary from one person to another, but the general consensus is that it can make life pretty unbearable at times.

With falling Oestrogen levels, Tinnitus is quite a common symptom of the Menopause but often lots of GP's don't make the connection. Apparently, Oestrogen underpins signaling from the ears to the brain and these falling levels could be responsible for mixing up the sounds being communicated between the two and cause the inner ear noise! But all is not lost, for some women Tinnitus may temporarily be caused by hormone levels fluctuating, and some studies have shown that in time the noises can disappear altogether or reduce in level.

The Best Help for Menopause Tinnitus:

Changing your diet, doing exercise and making some lifestyle changes are key to helping with Menopausal Tinnitus. Being in good shape inside and out is crucial to deal with this horrible Menopausal symptom. There are currently no remedies or drugs to cure this or operations to correct it, but you can take medication to deal with the sleep depravation that is often a huge problem with Menopausal Tinnitus. Audiologists may be able to find strategies to help you cope with and live with this debilitating symptom.

Natural Remedies to Try:

- Zinc – If you have age related Tinnitus, Zinc has been indicated in trials to help.
- Gingko Biloba – This can be good for circulation problems, especially if your Tinnitus is due to circulatory issues.

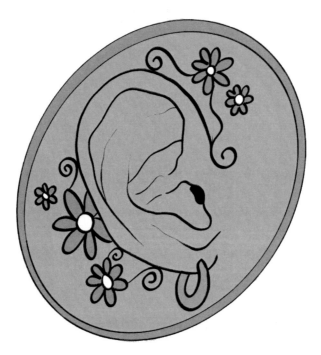

- B12 Vitamins – Tinnitus has been linked to a deficiency in B12.

Other things to avoid, to help with Tinnitus:

There can be a small increased risk of smokers developing Tinnitus, so avoid smoking. Foods that can exacerbate Tinnitus include salt, sodium and sugar, so avoid these too, also swapping your caffeine for a decaffeinated beverage, can help to settle symptoms of Tinnitus as caffeine keeps you awake at night too, so this will help with sleep.

Wellbeing to help with Tinnitus:

Keeping as healthy as possible may lessen your chances of suffering with Tinnitus. Our Adrenal glands pump out stress hormones which can make Tinnitus worse, but exercising helps flush out excess stress hormones, and can act as a massive distraction from worrying about Tinnitus.

Try relaxation techniques, white noise apps and sleep remedies to aid better sleep, these may help to get you off to sleep in the first place. Sleep deprivation has a huge impact on health but even more so for those suffering with Tinnitus.

Alternative Therapies:

I have been told by a few friends that have had Menopausal Tinnitus, that Acupuncture is definitely worth trying.

Aromatherapy, and Essential Oils have been used for many years to help with the treatment of Tinnitus. Aromatherapy can aid in relaxation and the use of Essential Oils may lessen the intensity of Tinnitus.

See Your GP/Doctor:

Most women who suffer with Menopausal Tinnitus are aged 40 – 60 and it is normally associated with hormone imbalances, but there could be other causes including heart disease, reactions to medications, or sweeteners. Always speak to your GP to rule out anything more sinister. Sometimes they will refer you for CBT (Cognitive Behavioral Therapy), which can help with the way you feel and cope with Tinnitus.

I hope this has given you an insight into another bizarre symptom of The Menopause!

Clumsiness and Bruising

For me, this first happened when I caught my hand on a table in a restaurant, and the result the next day looked horrendous! Yes, it hurt a bit at the time but NOTHING like the huge bruise I had on the whole of my arm the next morning! I seemed to be covered in bruises a lot of the time and often had no idea where they had come from! I had realized how clumsy I had become, but often put that down to my joint problems, I certainly had never been a clumsy person before, but walking into a door frame and misjudging where doors, cupboards and handles were, became a regular occurrence. I did not think much about it really until a few friends commented, and said they too had some huge bruises and had no idea as to why.

After looking into this (and actually feeling better about it after I had) I will let you into a few obvious but not so obvious reasons that I found!

Apparently, its all down to the falling of Oestrogen and Progesterone levels in the body. Often these two combined losses can cause a huge lack of concentration and make you feel giddy or have dizzy spells. Your lack of ability to judge distances and becoming more accident prone, are often caused by the diminishing of these hormones, and in some cases, minor car accidents and bangs due to lack of judgment and concentration can happen!

I never knew that falling Oestrogen levels could also affect your eyesight, so remember ladies to have regular eye tests, especially if you are beginning to squint more and can't see what you used to be able too!

As we get older our skin naturally begins to thin but as the Oestrogen levels drop this can get worse, so we don't have enough cushioning to protect us from those knocks and bumps, hence the huge bruises!

I am told it is all about balancing your hormones! Regular exercise is important as our bones can become weaker during this time, Yoga and Pilates are very good and help with balance. This is a major problem for some women as bad balance can cause them to trip and fall, and often is the reason the elderly are severely injured when they fall, mainly caused by their inability to balance.

Drinking lots of water is good for concentration, staying hydrated is so important for many issues caused by the Menopause and can aid with getting rid of headaches and feeling dizzy.

Being clumsy is not your fault and stress can also make you

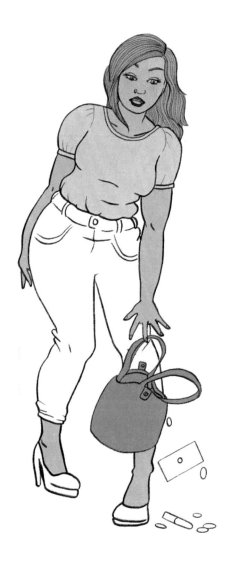

more prone to knocking things over and spilling things, it's a bit of a viscous circle, as the more you worry about being clumsy the more stressed you become. It is one of the side effects of the Menopause that should diminish as time goes by.

Some supplements can help with bruising, one friend of mine swears by Arnica, she says it stops her from bruising as badly. Vitamin A and C, and Bromelein (which is found in Pineapples) can help with healing too.

If you bruise easily it is also worth following these steps, apply pressure straight away, ice the area now and then, you can always use a light covering of makeup if necessary.

> Menopause isn't just about hot flushes and HRT! There are over 100 hormones in our bodies that can get out of balance and cause symptoms. It's vital to adapt your diet and lifestyle - not only to regain balance and improve your symptoms, but to focus on optimal health as you age.

Nicki Williams
(Founder of Happy Hormones for Life)

Itchy Skin

Hormone changes that occur during the Menopause can lots of issues and another very common one is Itchy Skin. This is also known as Pruritus and can start as early as the beginning of the Menopause (Perimenopause) and continues shortly after Menopause. With Oestrogen being related to the production of Collagen and the production of natural oils that keeps our skin moisturized, it is this that causes the skin to become thin and dryer and become itchy.

The most likely places on your body to become itchy are;

- Face
- Arms
- Legs
- Neck
- Chest
- Back
- Vagina

Your skin can also start suffering from conditions you have never suffered with before, including acne, rashes, wrinkling and change in pigmentation. Some women may experience tingling or numbness and pins and needles and lots of women seem to suffer from 'Formication' which is a type of Paresthesia, which is a feeing of insects crawling up your skin!

What you can do;

- Speak to your GP if your symptoms persist or last for 3 or 4 days or more, they may take some blood to rule out any other conditions. Sometimes medical intervention is needed if your condition is unbearable, or the skin is red and inflamed.
- Keep your skin well moisturised and use a good quality moisturiser as this will hold on to any water on the skin's outer layer and help stop the skin drying out.
- Use Aloe Vera or Calamine Lotion on any areas that are causing you discomfort.
- Vitamin C is incredibly important in the creation of collagen in the skin and aids skin repair and prevents itchy and dry skin too. A good quality supplement or eating foods with plenty of Vitamin C (most citrus fruits) is key.
- Some Herbal supplements like Maca Root and Dong Quai have been linked to aiding skin dryness too.
- HRT (Hormone Replacement Therapy) is quite popular in treating this condition and speaking to your GP might be a good idea to weigh up your options.

Preventing Itchy/Dry skin;

A few steps you can take to prevent or reduce your risk of dry/itchy skin are…

- Eating a healthy balanced diet and drinking lots of water to keep hydrated and the skin moisturised and supple.

- Taking good quality supplements has been shown to have great improvements on the skin, they include: Omega-3 fatty acids, Vitamin C, Primrose Oil and Collagen Peptides.
- Do not bath or shower in hot water as it takes the oils out of the skin, use lukewarm or cool water instead and do not use harsh soaps and perfumed products.
- Avoid smoking and alcohol which can both be very drying to the skin.
- Wear sun-cream daily if you are going outside.
- Take regular exercise.
- Get plenty of sleep.

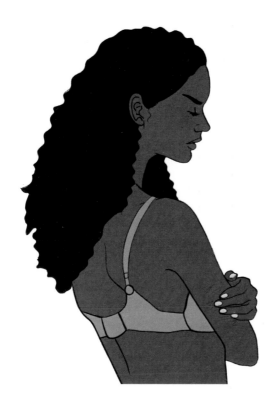

Genital Itching;

With the skin around the Vagina thinning, many women notice they are prone to itching (Vaginal Itching is called Vulvar Pruritus) this may occur more often if you experience vaginal dryness. With lowering Oestrogen levels this makes all the tissues around the Vagina and Vulva thinner and can make them very itchy and painful, it can also make sex more painful too. Always see your GP with any of these issues and of course any irregular bleeding.

Other factors to consider with Itchy and Dry Skin:

- Allergies
- Anxiety
- Hot Weather
- Cold Weather
- Smoking
- Alcohol
- Perfumed Products
- Eczema
- Psoriasis

Itchy skin is often a symptom of the Menopause and in time may subside after the Menopause has ended, a few lifestyle changes can help the severity of the itching. There are many different home remedies and supplements you can try too, but always see your medical professional if you are unsure or the symptoms get worse.

Panic Disorder and Irregular Heartbeat

Panic Attacks/Disorder

It is a turbulent time going through the Menopause for most women, with hormone levels dropping quickly and periods starting to slow down and eventually stopping altogether, we can experience some very unwelcome symptoms. Often the changes can affect the chemicals in your brain and that can have a huge effect on your mood. Going through Perimenopause and Menopause can cause lots of women to feel anxious or depressed, this is down to the changes in hormone levels but anything that is severe and ongoing should be investigated by your GP. With Oestrogen and Progesterone fluctuating in the body at this time, you can be left feeling anxious and depressed, but frequent panic attacks and high anxiety are common during the menopause, although they often go often once you are through Menopause.

What causes Panic Attacks during the Menopause?

The changes in hormone levels may influence the Neurotransmitters in the brain, and with additional factors such as sleep problems and hot flushes, this can lead to anxiety and low mood. Always speak to your GP if you find that you are feeling depressed daily, for more than a few weeks.

When to ask for help?

If your relationship is suffering or work becomes an issue because of anxiety or panic attacks and there is no other obvious problem there, it is a good idea to speak to your GP. If you are having thoughts of self-harm or negative thoughts for few weeks and cannot talk to anyone about the way you feel, either your GP or a therapist would be the best professionals to seek help from. Especially if you cannot understand or make sense of how you feel, do not leave it for weeks, get an appointment booked as soon as possible.

Treatment:

- HRT - (Hormone Replacement Therapy) can help with emotional symptoms as well as physical ones. It will not treat more severe mental health issues but can work well during the transition though the Menopause.
- Eating Healthily - this can change your mood and ease lots of Menopause symptoms.

- Sense of Achievement – Find a new hobby or interest that gives you purpose and set realistic goals.

- Exercise – This is great for changing your low mood into a positive one as lots of endorphins are released whilst exercising and therefore increase your mood.
- Talk to Friends or Family – Communication is important if you are feeling low, often just having a listening ear and someone with good positive advice can lift your mood instantly.
- Supplements – These can aid your mood, and you could be lacking in certain nutrients if your diet is not as healthy as it should be.

Irregular Heartbeat/Palpitations

I know some friends and a family member that have suffered with this and thought they were having a heart attack and were scared to death! Going through the Menopause can cause some strange symptoms, always seek advice from a medical professional if you develop these symptoms.

A fluttering or pounding heartbeat are called palpitations, they can happen if you are having a hot flush or can be tied to lots of other Menopause symptoms and happen for no reason. They feel like your heart is beating much faster than usual and can miss the odd beat or flutter, and you can sometimes feel the pounding in your throat or neck.

What can cause this?

The rise and fall of Oestrogen during the Menopause can cause heart palpitations or an irregular heart function. If you are having a hot flush your heart rate can increase its beats per minute, but it is not just this that can cause them. Stress, exercise, caffeine, alcohol, asthma, thyroid issues, low sugar, low blood pressure and dehydration can all cause palpitations.

When to seek help?

Suffering the odd time and on occasions lasting a few seconds is nothing to be too alarmed about but see your GP if you are concerned. If they last longer than a few minutes and get considerably worse over time then speak to a medial professional.

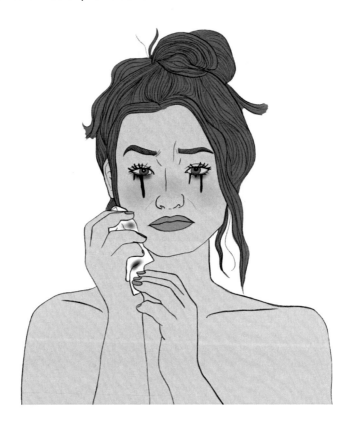

Always seek medical advice if you have shortness of breath, chest pain or feel dizzy or faint, as this could be a more serious issue that needs urgent medical attention.

Your GP may send you to a Cardiologist for further investigation and you may have to wear a heart monitor to check your heart function for a few days or so. It may be worth making a note of when these episodes happen, how long they last for and how it makes you feel.

Palpitations/Irregular heartbeat caused by the Menopause, is usually temporary and most women find their heart rhythm goes back to normal once they are post-Menopause. Your heart disease risk rises after the Menopause, some doctors think this is because Oestrogen was protecting the heart and once production is reduced, your risk of a heart attack or stroke goes up. Smoking, bad diet and alcohol increase your risks significantly, so now is the time to address those issues.

How can you avoid Palpitations/Irregular Heartbeat?

Avoid things that can make your heart race, this includes...

- Caffeine, chocolate, fizzy drinks, energy drinks and any other products that contain caffeine.
- Hot and spicy food.
- Smoking, alcohol.

Try relaxation techniques...

- Yoga/ Pilates.
- Reading a book.
- Meditation.
- Have a relaxing bath.
- Have a massage.
- Use breathing techniques.

Keeping your heart healthy before, during and after the Menopause is so important, eating healthy foods, exercising daily (even if it is a brisk walk), cutting back on salt and excess sugar and maintaining a healthy weight are all key to a healthy heart.

Hormone Replacement Therapy (HRT)

This has been a huge debate for many years now and I have spent a long time looking into the "Why's and Why not's" and the "pros and cons" of taking HRT and looking at the safety aspect of it too. Over a decade ago now there were massive headlines in the papers linking HRT to Breast Cancer and overnight women stopped taking it. Today less than 10% of women take HRT, and as one of the most effective treatments for most symptoms I am flabbergasted that we have all been given false information, and for so long!

• The WHI (Women's Health Initiative) Study.

The trial that was carried out 20 years ago was to look at the risks and benefits of older women taking HRT. Most of the women were an average age of 63, (women normally take HRT at a much younger age than that) so cannot be used to determine risks with women under that age and many were obese in this study too.

Two of the authors have recently published apologies for this misinterpretation of the study in the New England Journal Medicine.

• Suffering in Silence.

All the negative press and publicity led health professionals, doctors and GP's to be concerned about the potential risks of HRT, leading to thousands of women suffering horrendous effects of the Menopause and increased risk of Osteoporosis and Cardiovascular disease by not taking HRT.

• What is HRT.

HRT is a treatment that contains hormones, every woman is different and there are different ways you can take it (Will cover that below). They all contain Oestrogen, which you lose when your ovaries no longer make it after the Menopause.

• How can I Take It.

HRT comes in lots of different forms, you can take it in tablet form, patches, you can stick to your skin or gels you rub on your skin.

If you still have your womb – you will also need to take Progesterone. If you just take Oestrogen the womb lining can thicken and increase your risk of cancer of the Uterus. Some HRT products are combined and have both Oestrgoen and Progesterone.

If you're still having periods when you take HRT, you will be given an HRT that gives you regular periods. If a year has passed with no periods, or you have been taking HRT for more than a year, you will be given an HRT that will continue to not give you any periods.

Testosterone is another hormone that women produce, in lower amounts than men but it is still equally important. Low levels of Testosterone can cause women going through Menopause to have bad concentration, reduced libido, and no energy. This can be given as a cream that you can use daily.

• Benefits of taking HRT.

HRT can help with, if not improve massively, symptoms like Hot Flushes, Low Libido, Mood Swings, Night Sweats and even Bone Density improves with HRT, which is huge in the battle against Osteoporosis. The benefits and risks of HRT vary depending on age and any other health problems you have. ALWAYS speak to your GP about any concerns or issues you have. HRT has changed a lot over the years and taking it under 60 years old reduces your risks of Cardiovascular Disease. Starting HRT early can benefit your health, do not wait until it becomes unbearable. You can take HRT for as long as necessary and if you come off it, you pick up with your Menopause where it would have been had you not taken HRT, it does not delay your Menopause. Your quality of life is so important, and HRT can make you feel normal again and you can carry on living your life to the full again.

• HRT Risks.

For most women, the benefits of HRT outweigh the risks by a mile but so many women are badly informed and have been frightened into believing HRT is linked to Breast Cancer and is not safe to take. Like everything Menopause, EVERYONE is different and no ONE treatment fits all! It is so important to have a one to one with your GP or Menopause Specialist to discuss your risks, if any. Women who take some tablet forms of HRT have a small risk of developing a clot, but risks like obesity or having had a clot or stroke previously or smoking, are also risk factors that could make you more likely to suffer a clot or stroke. If you have suffered from these conditions before, you are more likely to be offered Oestrogen in a patch or gel form as opposed to tablet HRT.

With many women worrying about the link with HRT and Breast Cancer, some types of HRT do not increase the risk at all, and there may be a small number which do. The risk is so tiny it has been compared to the increased risk associated with drinking two small glasses of wine a night. There is still no study that proves that taking HRT can increase the risk of death from Breast Cancer.

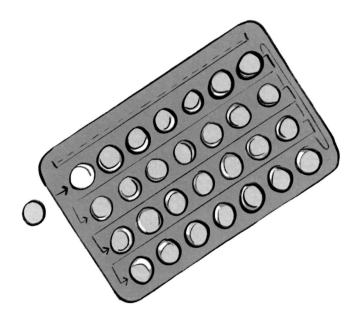

- ## HRT Side Effects.

These are usually very mild problems that occur in a few women, and usually happen in the first few months, and often settle down when the body gets used to the HRT. Initially, you may get some breast discomfort, feel a little nauseous, and patches may irritate the skin. Changing brand can often help or the type of HRT you are using.

Whatever your thoughts are on taking HRT, speak to your GP or Menopause Specialist about your options and symptoms. Most women will spend a third of their life Post-Menopausal and with 80% of women having several symptoms, lets not suffer in silence, there is help out there.

Men and the Menopause

I have received some lovely messages and emails from menopausal ladies asking me to write a bit about the menopause for their men!

Now I am no doctor and certainly no expert, but I have to say with some of the things I hear, there is a complete lack of information out there for women let alone men.

Even though roughly half the world's population is female, the menopause is very rarely spoken about or off, unless you're watching ITV at lunchtimes (when most people are at work) when those wonderful ladies at "Loose Women" talk about it. There has been some great programmes that have had us all talking about menopause but we need to make sure this doesn't go by the way side and we keep pushing to get this topic talked about and not the taboo subject it has been for many years.

The menopause is often hard for women to understand as there are hundreds of different symptoms! If Women find it hard to wrap their heads around and they go through it, there is no hope for men!

Some key facts that they should know...

Menopause starts with Perimenopause (before), then Menopause (during) and finally Postmenopausal (after) all these stages take many years and it's a long road for some.

It doesn't just happen it takes years to build up with sleep problems with anxiety, mood swings to name but a few.

Every woman experiences a completely different Menopause, So it's important for men to realise that women won't experience the same things in the same way.

Lots of men think that it must be better for women than their normal monthly period, but for most women they think it's like dementia and body hell put together.

There are lots of physical changes which can be very debilitating and hard to accept, hair changes, skin changes, mood swings, depression, anxiety, weight gain, low libido, brain fog, wanting to be alone and not venture out, and the list goes on.

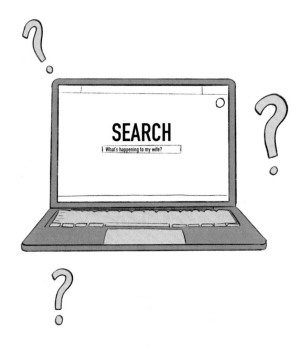

For women who have always been relatively slim suddenly a menopausal baby arrives! Whilst we all expect weight gain, suddenly it's very hard to make this excess weight budge. Some women find that just everything drops down, so maybe men need to accept this and hope that with lots of exercise, in time this will tone and firm up.

Another huge side-effect of the menopause is that a woman's metabolic rate slows down, and despite not eating any more, the increase around their middle still occurs. Going to the gym and exercising at least a few times a week and eating a sensible diet is essential at this time.

So gentlemen....

The advice is, when it comes to bad moods, try and understand that it isn't you. Sometimes treating her to a nice day out is a massive boost and shows you care.

When it comes to anything physical just remember that her body is changing and her confidence may have dropped as well as any drive she may have once had, just be respectful and be willing to talk about these things

Maybe share with her the differences you see in your own body i.e. your skin is more wrinkly, your waistline is bigger than it used to be and it's nice for her to know she's not the only one going through changes

Women lose lots of confidence at this debilitating and awful time, but to feel you're being supported on this long journey is a huge support to her. A surprise meal out or a treat shopping day or something she loves to do, can to her, make all the difference in the world.

I am hoping that women will show this book to their partners to help educate the male population on this topic!

Most women say their relationship has been affected and lots of women struggle to work.

What once was an unspoken topic is finally being accepted and talked about!

Thank you!

A huge thank you to my Parents Robin and June for supporting me throughout everything I do in life! Without your support I would not be publishing this book today! Also my sister Julie and her husband Steve, for their endless proofreading, tech support, belief and encouragement!

My heartfelt thanks to our wonderful illustrator Elle Freeman- without her talent, dedication and endless hours of work we would not have the amazing illustrations in this book that we do. Also a massive thank you to Darcie Venn for designing our front cover for us!

Many thanks also go to Andrew Bulpitt from Bulpitt print Ltd for finalizing and printing this book! We are truly grateful for your support and the time you spent on this for us!

Finally thank you to our readers! Without you supporting us and reading this book we wouldn't be able to keep pushing to spread the word about the menopause and help as many people as we do!

For more on The Menopause head over to clipboardclaire.com